Nursing OSCEs

Nursing OSCEs

A complete guide to exam success

EDITED BY

Catherine Caballero

Fiona Creed

Clare Gochmanski

Jane Lovegrove

All at the University of Brighton

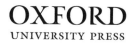

OXFORD

UNIVERSITY PRESS

OXFORD
UNIVERSITY PRESS

Great Clarendon Street, Oxford, OX2 6DP,
United Kingdom

Oxford University Press is a department of the University of Oxford.
It furthers the University's objective of excellence in research, scholarship,
and education by publishing worldwide. Oxford is a registered trade mark of
Oxford University Press in the UK and in certain other countries

Published in the United States of America by Oxford University Press
198 Madison Avenue, New York, NY 10016, United States of America

British Library Cataloguing in Publication Data
Data available

Library of Congress Cataloging in Publication Data
Data available

ISBN 978–0–19–969358–0

Preface

This book has been designed to help you develop the skills, knowledge and confidence to successfully complete a simulated (OSCE) examination. This book will provide you with an overview of the OSCE process. It will take you through an introduction to the use of simulation in nursing as a form of assessment of your clinical skills and will help you understand the OSCE process.

This book differs from other OSCE books as it specifically focuses on common skills that may be assessed via OSCEs in your university. It will enable you to revise for these specific skills and will help you to study appropriately for success.

Each chapter outlines the key revision required for your simulated examination, provides a step by step guide to the procedure, explains what the examiners are expecting of you, provides examples of OSCE criteria and common questions asked at each OSCE station and identifies top tips for helping you to pass your examination. The textbook is supported by a number of online resources available at the Online Resource Centre. These resources include colour step by step PowerPoint presentations of each skill, videos for selected skills and useful website addresses to help you fully prepare for your OSCE.

There are a number of people we would like to thank for their contributions to this book. Our thanks go to our colleagues at the University of Brighton and our local Trust Hospitals who have helped us with this book including Tina Attoe, Claire Cree, Paula Deamer, Kate Devis, Terry Stubbings and Sue Sully. Special thanks to Janette Grabham and production team for their assistance with video recording. We would also like to thank everyone at the Oxford University Press for their support and guidance in producing this book.

Thanks go to all the reviewers, academics, practitioners and students who offered their suggestions to improve this book. Their comments have been invaluable in this process.

We would also like to specially thank the first and second year students whose quotes are included (anonymously) throughout Chapter 14. These students were participants in Fiona's unpublished MSc research study exploring students' and lecturers' perceptions of the use of OSCEs in nursing education.

We sincerely hope you find this book valuable for your OSCE preparation and we wish you all success in passing your examinations.

Catherine Caballero, Fiona Creed,
Clare Gochmanski and Jane Lovegrove

Contents

About the editors and contributors

Editors

Dr Catherine Caballero DPhil, MSc, RN, PGCHSE, BSc (Hons), Dip Nursing. Senior lecturer at the University of Brighton. Catherine has a Doctorate of Philosophy from the University of Oxford. She has a background in surgical nursing, specializing in day surgery and in 1995 was appointed as the first laparoscopic nurse practitioner in the UK. Catherine's passion is in the development of clinical skills and her interests relate to clinical decision making, nursing knowledge, clinical skill development and mentorship and the support of learners in the clinical environment.

Fiona Creed MSc, BSc (Hons), RN. Senior lecturer at the University of Brighton. Fiona has a clinical background in general and neurological intensive care nursing and teaches acute clinical skills and post registration acute care nursing. Fiona is currently a PhD student at the University of Brighton where she is exploring clinical decision making during episodes of acute patient deterioration.

Clare Gochmanski is a skills laboratory technician at the University of Brighton. She is responsible for looking after five skills labs across the university sites assisting with simulation teaching, programming simulators and assisting with student skills practice session. Clare organizes and coordinates the OSCE examinations at the University.

Jane Lovegrove MSc, BEd, RNT, RN. Principal lecturer in clinical skills at University of Brighton. Jane's clinical background is in intensive care, cardiac surgery and coronary care. Her current clinical and educational interests are in grading clinical practice and using high fidelity simulation to assist students in clinical decision making.

Contributors

Tina Attoe RN, Dip Nursing, PGCHSE, MA. Senior Lecturer, School of Nursing and Midwifery, University of Brighton.

Clare Cree Dip Nursing, BSc (Hons), MSc. Lecturer Practitioner, School of Nursing and Midwifery, University of Brighton.

Paula Deamer RN, BSc (Hons), MA. Senior Lecturer, School of Nursing and Midwifery, University of Brighton.

Kate Devis RN, BSc (Hons), PGCE, MA. Previously Lecturer Practitioner for Clinical Skills between the University of Brighton and BSUH NHS Trust, and a Senior Lecturer at Mzuzu University, Malawi.

Terry Stubbings BA (Hons), RN (Adult), Dip Nursing (Lond.), PGCEA. Senior Lecturer, School of Nursing and Midwifery, University of Brighton.

Sue Sully MA BSc (Hons), PGDip, Dip Ed, RN, RNT. Senior Lecturer, School of Nursing and Midwifery, University of Brighton.

How to use this book

Nursing OSCEs: A complete guide to exam success has been specifically designed to help you revise and prepare for your OSCE as quickly and successfully as possible:

Key Revision

Everyone knows how busy life can be in the run up to exams, so this useful section quickly highlights the essential facts that you need to know for your OSCE.

> **Key revision for your simulated examination**
>
> *Systolic and diastolic values*
>
> Blood pressure is defined as the force exerted by blood against the walls of th contained (Docherty and McCallum 2009). A blood pressure measurement

Putting it all together for your OSCE

Step by step instructions clearly explain how to undertake a skill at the OSCE station. Accompanying photographs help you remember what to do.

> **Putting it all together!**
>
> You may be given a choice of manual or automated sphygmomanometer to use pressure, or you may be advised which device to use. Listen carefully to the inf by the examiner as an introduction to the assessment. An automated adult skills be used to represent a client – in both situations the examiner will check the r
> Ensure you use infection prevention strategies throughout the assess

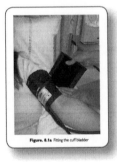

Figure. 8.1a Fitting the cuff bladder

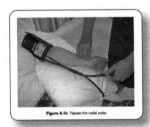

Figure 8.1b Palpate the radial pulse

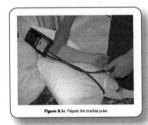

Figure 8.1c Palpate the brachial pulse

Video

When this video camera icon appears in the text a video of the skill is available on our online resource centre.

> Once your hands are sufficiently wet you should use the following techniques to clean every area of your hand.
>
> A video of this technique is included on the online resource centre **www.oxfordtext books.co.uk/orc/caballero**
>
> All steps of this process are vital and it is important that you fully understand and are able to demonstrate each step in your OSCE.

Examiners' marking criteria

Prepare for your OSCE by knowing exactly what the examiner expects of you ahead of the big day; you can use these checklists to practice with classmates and get feedback to improve your skills.

> **Examiners' marking criteria**
>
> Table 7.7 **Example of examiners' marking criteria**
>
> | Student's name and cohort year | |
> | --- | --- |
> | Expected performance criteria | Demonstrated Yes/No |
> | All observations | |
> | Student cleans hands (wash or alcohol gel). | |
> | Student approaches patient in a professional manner with introduction | |

Examiners' questions

You may be asked questions to assess your knowledge underpinning the OSCE stations. These examples are typical questions that examiners really do ask and answers are provided at the end of every chapter for quick revision.

Examiners' questions

You may be asked questions to assess your knowledge underpinning blood pr
Possible questions are provided in Box 8.3.

Box 8.3 Example of examiners' questions

1. What is the normal range for blood pressure in adults?
2. What does systolic pressure represent?
3. What does diastolic pressure represent?

Appendix: answers to examiners questions

1. What is the normal range for blood pressure in adults?
   100/60 mmHg – 140/90 mmHg
   Hypertension: systolic blood pressure ≥140 mmHg and diastolic blood pressure >
   Hypotension: systolic blood pressure <100 mmHg

Common errors in this examination

Avoid those classic mistakes by knowing what they are and consider our auther's advice to pass the first time

✗ Common errors at this station

As measuring blood pressure involves a number of important steps, and meas
ual sphygmomanometer involves technical skill, there are numerous possible p
may experience. The following section provides extra tips, but these are som
takes students may make:

Top tips

This quick list is perfect for consulting just before your OSCE.

✚ Top tips for passing this station

These are some suggestions to help you prepare and pass this station, based or
students' taking blood pressure measurements during OSCE.
   It can be difficult to remember the client when you are trying hard to reme
but do speak to the client when you are taking blood pressure measuremen
comfort.

About the online resource centre

The key to passing your OSCE is prepare, prepare, prepare—this book has a dedicated website to help you get started. These resources are freely available but are password protected. To access the resources simply visit the website and enter the followng username and password when instructed to in the book:

Username: caballero
Password: signpost

- Videos of key skills
- Powerpoints including colour photographs to aid revision
- Web links to evidence based guidelines so your knowledge is up-to-date
- Lecturer resources including tips and advice for running OSCEs

 You can find further advice and revision help for your OSCEs by going online now to
www.oxfordtextbooks.co.uk/orc/caballero/

PART I
Process and preparation

Chapter 1
An introduction to OSCE assessments

Fiona Creed

◎ Chapter aims

By the end of this chapter, you will understand:

- **OSCEs** and other types of simulated examinations,
- The background to simulated examinations,
- Why simulated examinations have been developed,
- The difference between **formative** and **summative** simulated examinations,
- Standardization of simulated examination,
- Aspects of skills assessed using simulation,
- The validity and reliability of simulated examinations.

➤ Introduction

It is likely that at some stage throughout your nursing programme you may be asked to attend a simulated examination. This often causes many students to panic a little as they are often unfamiliar with this type of examination and often unsure what this form of assessment involves and what they should expect. Simulated assessments are occurring with increasing frequency in many health care courses. They usually involve undertaking formal clinical examinations related to clinical skills outside of the clinical practice area. These examinations are referred to in a number of ways including OSCEs, university clinical assessments and clinical assessments. The key element common to all these assessments is that they use simulation in a non-clinical environment. That is to say the assessment occurs outside of a clinical environment—usually in a clinical skills room at your university. The purpose of this introductory chapter is to help you to understand:

- What is a simulated examination,
- The background to simulated examinations,
- Why simulated examinations have been developed,
- The difference between formative and summative simulated examinations,
- Standardization of simulated examination,
- Aspects of skills assessed using simulation,
- The validity and reliability of simulated examinations.

What is a simulated assessment/OSCE?

Within health care, several terms are used when discussing examinations using simulation and this may appear confusing. Therefore, to ensure consistency and to simplify discussion the term OSCE will be used throughout the book.

A simulated examination or simulated assessment is one that is examined using a simulated patient and/or a simulated situation. Assessors are provided with objective marking criteria and these criteria are used to judge the student's performance (Jones *et al.* 2010). Students are normally allocated a set amount of time to complete the assessment and they are provided with feedback in relation to their assessment. This is referred to as an OSCE (Objective Structured Clinical Examination) in several universities, although other terms may be used.

Whilst there are considerable variations, in the use of simulated examinations in health care it is important to acknowledge that common features exist. These common features include:

- Examinations which are held in a simulated environment usually within a university setting/university clinical skills room/simulation area.
- Examinations which use actors or other students/lecturers in the place of real patients.
- Examinations which usually adhere to university examination regulations.
- Assessors are usually university lecturers. Occasionally expert practitioners will be involved in the university assessments.
- Students are normally required to 'rotate' around a number of clinical assessment 'stations'. This allows the assessment of several skills during one examination.

Several health care professions now use simulated examinations including:

- Nursing
- Paramedics
- Physiotherapists

This type of assessment began in medicine where simulated examinations have been a common feature of clinical assessment throughout the UK for several years.

Historical development of examinations using simulation

OSCE examinations were first developed in 1979 by Harden and Gleeson for the assessment of clinically focused skills in medical students. In the original development students rotated around 20–30 stations and would spend 5–10 minutes at each station either performing one skill or writing answers to an exam.

Harden and Gleeson (1979) felt that this approach was more reliable than traditional forms of assessment. It also places emphasis on the importance of developing effective clinical skills.

The popularity of the assessment of clinical skills using simulation rapidly spread throughout medical schools in the UK and now the majority of medical schools test their students using these methods. Because of the widespread adoption of this assessment method there are similarities between what is assessed and the structure of the assessment throughout medical schools in the UK. This has led to some standardization of what is assessed and how it is assessed.

Since this initial development in the UK the use of OSCEs to assess students has spread internationally and to other disciplines. They have been widely adapted in medicine to assess clinical competence and modified to suit local conditions. In the last decade the use of OSCE as an assessment tool has become very popular in nursing and allied professions.

Why have simulated examinations been developed?

Initial simulated examinations were designed to allow the assessment of clinical skills in a safe environment away from the clinical area where mistakes in assessment and diagnosis would not be detrimental to patient care (Bloomfield *et al.* 2010). They were initially derived to be an assessment strategy but are more importantly viewed as a learning tool whereby the student is provided with objective, expert clinical feedback to allow the student to learn from the assessment and improve their practice.

However, alongside the need for learning from clinical assessment, several other factors have encouraged the development of the simulated examinations across all health care courses. These factors include:

Professional regulation   Some regulatory bodies, most notably the Nursing and Midwifery Council (NMC), have made explicit the need for simulated examinations during nursing pre-registration programmes. Whilst the NMC does acknowledge the need for the majority of skills to be assessed in practice it has begun to acknowledge the importance of assessment through simulation. The essential skill clusters (NMC 2007) clearly identify the need for skills to be assessed using simulation prior to admission to branch. The only area that this explicitly relates to currently is assessment of aseptic technique, where the NMC states that this must be assessed through simulation by the end of year 1. The NMC may make further recommendations in relation to simulated examinations in the future.

The inclusion of skills that require assessment using simulation has meant that most universities that provide pre-registration nursing programmes are required to include these examinations as part of the student nurse's educational programme.

Patient safety   Health care is becoming increasingly litigious and the need to protect the patient and maintain patient safety is clearly paramount. Some educationalists feel it is more appropriate to allow the student time to learn practice and be assessed in a simulated environment prior to experience with patients in a clinical area. These educationalists acknowledge that there is a need for students to be assessed in clinical practice as well, but maintain that practice and assessment outside of the clinical area using simulation will enhance real clinical experience.

Drive for objective assessment   Recent educational studies, most notably Duffy's research (2004), have identified inconsistencies in clinical assessment. These inconsistencies have affected the objectivity of clinical assessments and it is argued that several students have passed clinical skills assessments where they perhaps should have failed. Other factors may also make objective assessment of clinical skills difficult. These include lack of time or resources for clinical assessment, interruption of the business of ward areas, increasing scarcity of appropriate clinical placements and the limited opportunity to assess some skills in some clinical areas. It is also acknowledged that care of the patient should always take priority over assessment of the student and in some very busy areas this does reduce the time professionals have for student assessment.

Educational establishments' valuing of clinical skills   The use of simulated examinations in health care requires a huge investment of resources by educational establishments. The resources required include:

- Setting up the examination,
- Running the examination,
- Providing feedback,
- Post assessment counselling/developing action plans.

Investment in these costly resources highlights the value that universities attach to the development of clinical skills.

Formative versus summative clinical examination

Simulated examinations are usually referred to as being a summative or formative examination. This educational terminology often confuses students and registered nurses alike so it is vital to clarify the type of examination being assessed.

Summative examination   This is an examination that the student must pass in order to progress in their chosen career. These summative exams are typically held in 'key stages' of the student's course. For example, in nursing, summative examinations may be held prior to admission to the branch programme at the end of the first year or prior to admission to the professional register at the end of the final year. Students are normally allowed up to three sometimes four attempts to pass a summative examination, although this, of course, depends on the university's examination regulations.

Formative examination   This is an examination designed to provide the student with constructive objective feedback about the area being assessed. There is not normally a requirement for the student to pass a formative examination although some universities may insist that the student retakes the examination to demonstrate learning as a result of the initial examination. Most universities will use formative examinations as an opportunity to develop an action plan with the student that will enable them to build upon and enhance their skill/knowledge.

Standardization of skills assessed using simulated examinations

It was highlighted earlier that there does appear to be some standardization of simulated examinations in medicine and medical students can expect to sit very similar types of simulated examinations throughout the UK.

However, in other health care professions the type of examination and the subject of the examination may vary greatly between institutes and there is currently very little standardization in the UK. This reflects the early stage of development of simulated examinations in other health care professions. It is expected that some guidance may be provided by regulatory bodies, e.g. the NMC, but at the moment this has not yet happened.

Which aspects of skills are assessed?

Again there is great variation in which aspects of skills are assessed. This varies between universities and between health care professions. In general, simulated examinations will assess the performance of a skill and professional attributes associated with that skill and may or may not assess the knowledge related to the skill.

Box 1.1 **Remember**

You are strongly advised to discuss the type and nature of simulated examination that is used in your university with the lecturers that are involved with simulated examinations. This book will provide a general overview and general guidance in relation to simulated examinations in health care with a particular emphasis on pre-registration nursing. Examples of skills likely to be assessed are included in Table 1.1.

Table 1.1 **Examples of skills in nursing that may be tested via OSCE**

Nursing	What is involved
Physiological measurements	Recording of vital signs. These may be recorded individually at separate stations or recorded all together as you would in clinical practice .This should include: • Blood pressure, • Temperature, • Respirations, • Pulse, • Oxygen saturations (see Chapter 7).
Aseptic technique	You will be asked to demonstrate the use of an aseptic technique. This may involve undertaking a wound dressing on an actor or simulation manikin or using another situation, e.g. urinary catheterization that requires you to use an aseptic technique (see Chapter 6).
Medication administration	You will be required to administer medication, usually oral medication to an actor. You will be required to demonstrate an underpinning knowledge of all of the safety aspects relating to medication administration (see Chapter 11).
CPR	You will be asked to demonstrate effective resuscitation principles on a manikin. This may be a child/baby or an adult. You will be expected to use the current Resuscitation Council (UK) Guidelines (see Chapter 13).
Drug calculation	You will be asked to correctly undertake drug calculation. Whilst this will be tested to some extent in drug administration, you will be expected to perform complex drug calculations. This may be a computer test or a paper test (see Chapter 10).
Assessment of a sick patient	You will be asked to systematically assess a patient. It is likely that the patient will be a simulation manikin but actors may be used. You will be expected to follow a logical assessment process and identify any changes in your patient quickly and appropriately. This is a complex skill and is usually tested in your final year (see Chapter 12).

Performance of skill   The performance of a skill is an essential element to all simulated examinations. Some simulated examinations will only assess the ability to correctly perform a skill. This is known as assessment of the psychomotor elements of the skill. The university may test underpinning knowledge that relates to the skill by using another examination format, e.g. multiple choice tests.

Professional attributes   Most simulated examinations will assess whether the skill is performed in a professional manner. This may involve assessing whether the student is attired professionally, communicates with the patient effectively, understands the limitations of their ability, understands the need to appropriately approach the patient and maintains an appropriate attitude to the patient and/or situation.

Box 1.2 **Remember**

You are strongly advised to discuss what parts of the skill are being assessed in the simulated examination that is used in your university with the lecturers that are involved with examinations. The lecturers will identify which areas are being assessed in each simulated examination.

Knowledge related to the skill   Many universities fundamentally believe that skills and knowledge are so inextricably linked that there is a need to assess these together. In these examinations it is likely you will be asked a series of questions that will demonstrate your understanding of the theory or knowledge related to that skill.

Validity/reliability of simulated examinations

Many students worry that their examination will be difficult and that some examiners will be stricter than others when marking the examinations. All examinations are rigorously tested to ensure that the examination measures what it is intended to do (validity) and that it is a fair and equitable experience (reliability).

Validity   All universities will have invested a considerable amount of time ensuring that the examination does test the associated skill accurately. To this end most examination marking tools are tested time and time again and refined until the examiners are sure that the examination can assess that skill appropriately. In addition to this, most universities insist that those assessing the skill are clinical experts and these lecturers/clinical staff may be required in some universities to be assessed using simulated examinations before they are permitted to be an examiner for that particular skill.

Reliability   Again universities have several systems in place to determine that simulated examinations are as fair and objective as possible. Some universities use advanced statistical analysis of each station and of each examiner and each examiner is given a score representing the overall fairness, parity and objectivity. This system ensures that examiners are consistently fair and subjectivity is avoided.

   You must therefore be reassured that you will be assessed fairly by nurses or lecturers who have expertise in teaching or undertaking the clinical skills they are assessing. The use of objective criteria will ensure you are assessed in exactly the same manner as the other students in your cohort or group.

How can this book help you?

Having completed the action points (see Box 1.3) it is advisable to continue reading through the following chapters, as your time allows. The next two chapters in the book will help you to understand more details about OSCE assessments:

- **Chapter 2** will provide an overview of 'typical OSCE stations' to enable you to understand how your OSCE assessment may be undertaken.
- **Chapter 3** will provide you with some advice on how you may begin to prepare yourself for your OSCE assessment.

Once you understand exactly what an OSCE involves and how you can prepare, you are advised to read the following chapter or chapters that relate to your own OSCE:

- **Chapters 4–13** will provide detail related to specific OSCE assessments. These subjects have been chosen as a representation of skills your university may assess using an OSCE assessment. It is most unlikely that you will be assessed on all of these skills so you may just wish to initially concentrate on the skills your own university assesses. However the other chapters will be useful for assessment of these skills in practice.
- These chapters have been carefully planned to ensure that they each include:
  - Key revision for your OSCE assessment,
  - Step by step explanation of the skill you are being assessed on using evidence-based explanations for each step,
  - An example of an OSCE criteria grid for that skill,
  - Common mistakes made at that OSCE station and how to overcome these,
  - Top tips for passing your OSCE,
  - Reading/reference lists that you may wish to refer to,
  - Links to electronic material available on the OSCE book website see **www.oxfordtextbooks.co.uk/orc/caballero/**.

Throughout the skills-focused chapters there are some common themes that examiners will be assessing you on and emphasis will be placed on these important aspects. These include:

- Professional attitude,
- Communication with the patient and other staff,
- Ability to undertake the skill effectively,
- Knowledge related to the skill,
- Ability to maintain **infection control,**
- Documentation throughout the process.

These are all important features and will be common aspects of the assessment. It is important that you pay attention to these areas when preparing for and undertaking your OSCE.

The final chapter, **Chapter 14**, focuses on the use of reflection in the OSCE assessment practice. This is of particular use in formative and summative assessments as you may wish to reflect upon the areas you have done well in and begin to explore how you may improve on aspects of the assessment that you felt could be better.

What now?

At this stage, it will be useful to develop your own personal study plan which may include:

- Checking that you understand what an OSCE may involve. You may wish to read around the subject of OSCE and it may be useful to review some of the references in the reference list if you would like more detailed explanations. You may wish to utilize the personal study plan to identify what you have learnt from this chapter and what you need to plan to do next.
- Discussing with your own university's clinical skills team which OSCE you will be expected to undertake during your nursing programme.
- Reviewing the skills chapters that will be useful either in your OSCE or in clinical practice.

Box 1.3 **Personal study plan**

Five important things I have learnt from reading this chapter

Plan for future reading/study/revision

Online resource centre

You can find further advice and revision help for your OSCEs by going to online now to see www.oxfordtextbooks.co.uk/orc/caballero/.

≋ References

Bloomfield, J., Pegram, A. and Jones, C. (2010). *How to pass your OSCE: a guide to success in nursing and midwifery.* Harlow: Pearson Education.

Doran, T. and O'Neil P. (2002). *Core clinical skills for OSCEs in medicine.* London: Churchill Livingstone.

Duffy, K. (2004). *Failing Students.* London: Nursing & Midwifery Council.

Harden, R.M. and Gleeson, F.A. (1979). Assessment of clinical competence using an OSCE. *Medical Education* 13:41–54.

Jones, A., Pegram, A. and Fordham, C. (2010). Developing and examining an objective structured clinical examination. *Nurse Education Today* 30:137–141.

Nursing and Midwifery Council (2007). *Essential skills clusters.* London: Nursing and Midwifery Council.

Chapter 2
Overview of the OSCE station
Fiona Creed

Chapter aims

This chapter will help the reader understand:

- What to expect from an OSCE,
- How simulated exams are organized,
- The examination environment,
- The role of the patient and examiner,
- The structure of a simulated examination,
- The timing of a simulated examination,
- Examination regulations,
- Top tips for understanding the structure of your own examination.

Introduction

Student health care practitioners are often apprehensive about simulated examinations as they have never undertaken an examination like this before and often do not know what to expect. The purpose of the chapter is to explore the OSCE process and help you to understand and plan for your own OSCE.

Organization of simulated examinations

OSCE examinations may be organized very differently depending upon the subject of the examination and your own university's preference. Most simulated examinations are held in clinical skills rooms or simulation suites at the student's university campus. Very occasionally they may be held off site at another location, e.g. a hospital teaching room.

The examination structure may vary dramatically (Bloomfield *et al.* 2010) and may be:

- Multiple short stations,
- Complex single stations,
- Unmanned station.

Multiple short station OSCEs

These are also known as 'short case' OSCE stations. A typical short station OSCE will involve the student health care practitioner 'rotating' around a number of different stations. It is likely that within each examination room several skills will be assessed at any one time and part of the assessment will involve moving from station to station to ensure that students complete all skills/knowledge assessments that are required (see Fig. 2.1). This format allows examiners to assess a range of skills during one simulated examination period (Ahuja 2009). The number of stations will depend upon the university's examination structure but it may be that there are up to five stations to attend. Some universities ask students to rotate around more than this (in some occasions up to 20). This type of OSCE is very common in pre-registration nursing OSCEs (Bloomfield et al. 2010).

Simulated examinations may be held in one room or students may be required to move from room to room to ensure all skills are assessed.

Complex single station OSCEs

This type of OSCE is usually used to examine the more complex skills and may be used in the final year to test more complicated skills such as assessment of the sick patient. You should be aware that you may also be asked to undertake OSCE in your post-registration nurse education. Most post-registration OSCEs use this approach as they are likely to want to test competency in the integration of a number of skills, e.g. neurological examination in a physical assessment course. It is common for knowledge to be tested in this sort of OSCE.

Unmanned station

This may be a component of multiple short station OSCEs. Some universities will require you to complete either a paper or online assessment examination that tests your knowledge as well as your ability to undertake a skill. This station is usually still timed so you have to be careful with your time management but there is usually no one present at this station. Some universities may also ask you to stay at a waiting station whilst you wait for your colleagues to finish their OSCE. If this approach is used you are not allowed to discuss the OSCE with other students (discussion

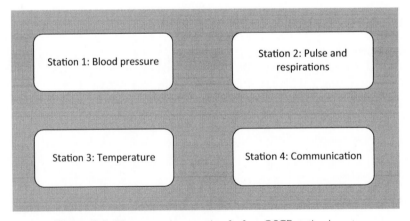

Figure 2.1 Diagrammatic example of a four OSCE station layout

during the course of the OSCE process is often unhelpful as it only serves to make the other students nervous!).

Layout of the OSCE station

At each OSCE station the student will have one particular simple or complex skill to complete. Some universities split skills down into very small components, e.g. hand washing only. Other universities may wish to create a more realistic assessment and require the student to complete all **physiological measurements (blood pressure, pulse,** respiration, **oxygen saturation** and temperature) within one station. It is important that prior to attending the examination students find out which sort of approach has been adopted by the university. Regardless of type of approach the layout of the simulated examination station will be similar (see Fig 2.2 and Fig 2.3).

Each station will usually include:

- A patient,
- An examiner,
- A skill to complete,
- The necessary equipment to complete the skill,
- Documentation if required, e.g. observation chart,
- Filming equipment if used,
- Infection control equipment, e.g. hand gel, aprons, gloves.

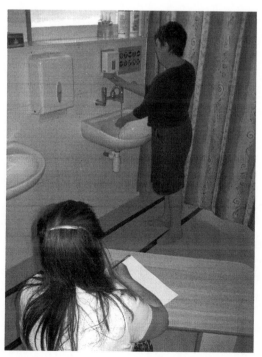

Figure 2.2 Hand washing

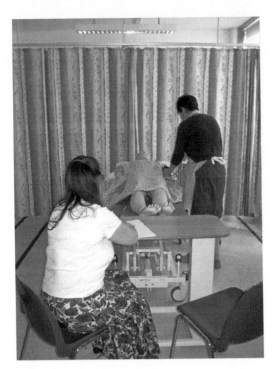

Figure 2.3 Physiological measurement station

Roles and responsibilities

The role of the patient

The patient may be required at some stations, e.g. for communication or physiological measurements. Other stations, e.g. hand washing, may not have a patient present. At some stations, e.g. injection technique, you may only have a model of the skin. The role of the patient may be played by:

- Another lecturer,
- A member of staff from a local NHS Trust,
- A fellow student,
- A patient volunteer,
- A simulated patient (see Fig. 2.4).

The student is expected to treat the patient as they would in clinical practice. This is to ensure that the student can be assessed for appropriate communication skills, interaction with the patient, and professional attitude. It is also to ensure that the student considers legal issues, e.g. gaining consent prior to treatment/assessment, and remembers to follow universal precautions to prevent the spread of infection to the patient.

It is sometimes difficult but essential to treat this role play patient as a real patient in clinical practice. The role play patient is often involved in marking or judging attitude and communication skills of the student and will often be involved in assessing how well the student has performed.

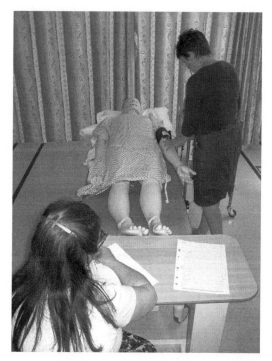

Figure 2.4 A simulated patient

Box 2.1 Remember

You will be assessed on your interpersonal skills and how you interact with the patient. This is often a difficult part of the assessment when you are nervous. At each station where a patient is used you must:

- Introduce yourself to the patient,
- Communicate throughout the station in a professional manner,
- Gain consent for everything you are doing,
- Explain everything you are going to do in terms that the patient will understand,
- Check the patient's understanding prior to the procedure,
- Always ensure your patient's dignity and privacy are respected (it is easy to forget to draw the curtains in an artificial situation!),
- Maintain the safety of the patient at all times,
- Prevent the spread of infection to your patient (remember to decontaminate your hands!).

The role of the examiner

The examiner is present to assess the student and will often be a lecturer that students are familiar with or may be an expert clinician or another lecturer from the university. The role of the examiner is to:

- Explain the station to the student (see examples in Table 2.1),
- Assess the student throughout the examination using the assessment tool,
- Provide feedback to the student (either at the end of the examination (formative) or by written communication (summative)).

Table 2.1 **Examples of an examiner's explanation of an OSCE station to a student**

OSCE station	Examiner's explanations
Blood pressure	I would like you to record this patient's blood pressure and document it on this observation chart.
Full set of observations	I would like you to record a full set of observations on this patient. When the observations are complete I would like you to calculate the MEWS (Modified Early Warning Score).
Hand washing	I would like you to demonstrate effective hand washing.
Recognition of the sick patient	Examiner A will provide you with a handover for this patient and I would like you to systematically assess him/her following the **ALERT® (Acute Life-Threatening Events Treatment and Recognition)** protocol.
Aseptic technique	This patient's dressing needs changing. I would like you to review her care plan and dress the wound, following the wound care plan, using an aseptic technique.

It is unlikely that the examiner will engage in any communication with the student other than to issue instructions for that station and this may make you feel nervous, but remember the same instructions will be given to each student to ensure parity of communication (Jones *et al.* 2010). It would not be fair to provide one student with complex instructions and another with very little detail and this is why these standardized instructions are used.

Remember to ensure you understand what is being asked of you at each station; you can, of course, ask the examiner to repeat the instructions if you are at all unsure.

If any problems occur during the assessment process the examiner may stop the examination. This is unlikely but may happen if you are causing pain or potential harm to the patient. One common error, for example, is to leave the blood pressure cuff fully inflated for a long time whilst attempting to hear the **systolic pressure** when recording a manual blood pressure. The examiner may ask that you let the cuff down and rest the 'patient' if they appear to be in any discomfort.

The examiner will be looking for safe and competent practice. Doran and O'Neil (2002) suggest that this may be reflected in:

- Approach,
- The fluency of skills performance,
- Dexterity in performing the skill,
- Application of knowledge,
- Clear communication.

Assessment

Assessment criteria

The examiner will be assessing the performance of that skill against predefined criteria. He or she will most likely be marking an **assessment criteria** sheet as you progress through that station. Some students are alarmed at this, especially if the examiner appears to be writing a lot. Do not worry about this. Throughout the skill the examiner will assess the student against predefined criteria that will enable an overall assessment of the competence at the end of your examination (Ahuja 2009). In some examinations 'red flags' may be used; these are points that the students must cover in order to pass that skill, e.g. appropriate **hand decontamination** if patient contact is required. Some universities have particular stations that must be passed in order for you to achieve an overall pass grade in your OSCE.

Assessment criteria will vary from university to university and it is good practice for the examiners to allow the students to see the marking criteria prior to the examination to ensure that they are aware of the criteria that they are being assessed against. Students should also be notified of any red flag criteria (criteria that must be demonstrated in order to pass).

An example of marking criteria is shown in Table 2.2, but it is stressed that this may vary greatly and students should familiarize themselves with the marking grid that is to be used.

Box 2.2 **OSCE tip**

Your tutors will have already highlighted the red flags to you in your OSCE preparation sessions. If there are going to be any red flags remember to record these in your revision notes so that you do not forget them on the day of your OSCE.

How will the examiner mark the examination?

This will be very dependent upon the marking style of the university and it is vital that students are aware how the examination will be graded. There are several different methods that may be used and it is essential that you understand which marking criteria your own university is using:

- **Total mark awarded:** Some universities will provide a grade for your OSCE performance. Where this approach is used the examiner will award you a total mark depending on how well you have performed aspects of the OSCE. You may be awarded marks for aspects of the OSCE, e.g. interpersonal skills, professional attitude, and demonstration of skill and associated knowledge. Alternatively each component will be awarded a score. Where this approach is used each part of the examination will be awarded a mark and the mark awarded will be a sum of these marks—it may be calculated as a percentage of the total score. This approach is often used in universities that recognize the importance of grading the clinical component of nursing alongside the academic work.
- **Pass/fail:** Some examinations will simply be marked as a pass or a fail and this is perhaps the simplest form of marking (Rushforth 2007). The OSCE checklist will be broken down into action observed/not observed. Failure to complete all of the components of the OSCE will result in a fail grade award.
- **Global mark:** Some examiners give a global grade for the station. In this case examiners will be asked to identify how well each component of the skill was performed and this provides a view of the quality of the skills performance (Rushforth 2007). Examiners will be asked to identify whether the skill performance was excellent/good/satisfactory/borderline/refer. It is likely that the examiners will have objective descriptors to help them differentiate between excellent and good. Other universities may use a Likert scale to determine global rating (see Fig. 2.5).

Table 2.2 **Example of examiners' marking criteria**

Student's name and cohort year	
Expected performance criteria	Demonstrated Yes/No
Student is wearing a uniform and is adhering to their local uniform policy.	
Hair that is longer than collar length is secured neatly.	
Student removes any rings/jewellery/watches.	
Nails are short/no nail varnish/no false nails/no nail jewellery.	
Student ensures any cuts/abrasions are covered.	
Student's arms are bare below the elbow.	
Taps are adjusted so water flow is steady and does not splash back.	
Student wets hands.	
Soap is applied and lather created.	
Student washes hands ensuring the thumbs, fingernails, fingertips, palms, backs of hands, between fingers and wrists are thoroughly washed. See RCN technique. If a single band ring is worn the student washes underneath and around it.	
Hands washed for at least 15 seconds.	
All soap is then rinsed off.	
Taps turned off using elbow/sensor.	
Hands are dried thoroughly on paper towel.	
Paper towel disposed of according to local policy (black bag).	

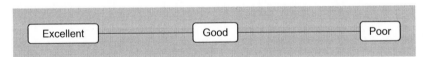

Figure 2.5 Likert scale

- **Combination approach:** Some universities may use pass/fail or grade criteria alongside a global rating scale (Rushforth 2007; Jones *et al.* 2010). This combined approach is thought to be a reliable and fair way of assessing students.
- **Red flag criteria met/unmet:** If red flag criteria are not met then the student will not be awarded a pass grade. Common red flag criteria often relate to important issues such as consent and infection control. These are sometimes overlooked in the stress of an OSCE examination but are essential components of effective patient care.

Timing within simulated examinations

Students are usually given a stated amount of time in which to complete each skill during a simulated examination. The timing of the examination is an important component as it is essential that each student is allowed to have the same amount of time for each station to ensure parity throughout the assessment.

Most examinations will commence with the examiner telling students when the assessment will begin. Students are usually also warned either 1 or 2 minutes before the end of the examination as well. This strict timing can often make the examination feel more stressful and increase anxiety. However, the examiners have usually carefully calculated how much time a practitioner at any given level should take to complete the assessment so students should not feel rushed in this situation.

Examination conditions

Simulated examinations are normally held under the university's examination regulations. This means that students are expected to adhere to examination rules and behave in accordance with these regulations. Most universities will require you to wear your uniform for the OSCE so remember to pack your uniform when preparing for the OSCE and allow plenty of time to change.

Filming

It may be a requirement for the examination to be filmed. The filming serves two purposes:

- It enables the external examiner to check simulated examinations as part of an examination board process. This is usually only done if the assessment is summative and if this is a requirement of your university.
- It enables the student to view their own performance and reflect back on the process as part of the learning from the simulation. This is normally only used if the examination is formative.

Where filming is used it is usually unobtrusive (cameras may be located in the ceilings of skills rooms/simulation suites). On some occasions other cameras will be used. Students may or may not be required to wear a microphone so that filming will include any verbal interactions throughout the examination.

Practice sessions

Some universities offer the opportunity for students to attend practice sessions and may schedule them into your student timetable. If optional practice sessions are offered students are strongly advised to attend as these will give the opportunity to experience a simulated examination prior to undertaking a more formalized assessment.

Top tips for preparing for OSCE examinations

Before the OSCE day:

- Familiarize yourself with setting and layout,
- Find out if you are required to wear your uniform,

- Find out how much time there is for each station/skill,
- Look at the marking criteria that is going to be used,
- Find out if there are any red flags in each exam,
- Find out how the exam will be marked,
- Attend any practice sessions that are offered,
- Recognize that you need to treat a patient (real or otherwise) as a patient,
- Find out if the simulation is to be assessed using a low/high fidelity manikin to avoid any shocks during the examination.

On the day of the OSCE:

- Act professionally throughout the examination,
- Do not expect to have the same relationship with the examiner during the exam as you do in every-day lectures,
- Communicate with the patient and examiner throughout the examination,
- Ensure that you leave the patient in a comfortable and safe position,
- Try to view the examination as a learning tool.

The next chapter will discuss how you can prepare yourself for the OSCE examination, but before moving on it may be a good idea to complete the checklist in Table 2.3 to ensure you are aware of everything that your own OSCE will include.

If you do not know the answers to any of these questions speak to a member of your university's skills/OSCE team who will be able to help and reassure you.

Table 2.3 **OSCE checklist**

Find out the following:	
• What sort of OSCE station will I be doing (single or multiple)?	
• What skills will be assessed?	
• Is there a knowledge assessment?	
• Are there any unmanned stations?	
• How will the stations be organized?	
• Who will be the patient (lecturer/patient/manikin)?	
• What criteria will I be assessed against?	
• Are there any red flags?	
• Are there any killer stations that I must pass?	
• How will the OSCE be marked (percentage mark, pass/fail, global mark)?	
• How much time will be allowed for each station?	
• What are the examination regulations for my OSCE?	
• Will I be filmed or required to wear a microphone?	
• Are there any practice sessions?	
• Can I practise with a group of friends?	
• Do I have any concerns that I need to discuss with the lecturers?	

Online resource centre

You can find further advice and revision help for your OSCEs by going online now to see **www.oxfordtextbooks.co.uk/orc/caballero/.**

References

Ahuja, J. (2009). OSCE: a guide for student practitioners. *Practice Nurse,* 37(1): 37–39.

Bloomfield, J., Pegram, A. and Jones, C. (2010). *How to pass your OSCE: a guide to success in nursing and midwifery.* Harlow: Pearson.

Doran, T. and O'Neil, P. (2002). *Core clinical skills for OSCE in medicine.* London: Churchill Livingstone.

Jones, A., Pegram, A. and Fordham-Clarke, C. (2010). Developing and examining an objective structured clinical examination. *Nurse Education Today,* 30: 137–141.

Rushforth, H. (2007). Objective structured clinical examination (OSCE): review of the literature and implications for nursing practice. *Nurse Education Today,* 27: 481–490.

Chapter 3
Preparation for the OSCE assessment
Fiona Creed

◎ Chapter aims

This chapter will provide an overview of general preparation required. This will include:

- Understanding how preparation will help you in your OSCE,
- Key revision strategies,
- Key practice strategies,
- Key points to help you.

➤ Introduction

The need to prepare adequately for any university examination is beyond refute and students may struggle with the OSCE assessment if they are unprepared or have unrealistic expectations of the OSCE process (Bloomfield *et al.* 2010). Adequate preparation will enable you to:

- Minimize any anxiety related to the examination,
- Understand the requirements of the OSCE,
- Facilitate accurate, systematic and timely performance of the OSCE,
- Enable you to give full justice to your professional ability.

OSCEs represent an important opportunity for you to further develop your nursing knowledge and skills. Effective preparation will give you a better opportunity to learn effectively from your OSCE and enable you to view the experience positively (see Chapter 14 Reflecting upon your OSCE).

Preparation for your OSCE will clearly be affected by your own learning style and where and how you study is likely to be adapted to suit your own learning needs. You may well have completed a learning style assessment quiz such as Honey and Mumford's (1986) at university; if not, you are able to access this online. It may be best to link your study for your OSCE to your learning style. Honey and Mumford (1986) identified several differing learning styles that are briefly described here. These include:

- Reflector: Tend to explore issues in depth before reaching a decision,
- Theorist: Logical and enjoy researching and using theory to enable understanding,
- Pragmatist: Like to apply things in practice and experiment with new ideas,
- Activists: Are open to new ideas and learn through experience alongside others.

Therefore you can use your understanding of your learning style to help plan how you may best revise/prepare for your OSCE. For example:

● Activist: May prepare best by practising for your OSCE with your colleagues and practising your OSCE in the skills room or in a group outside of university.
● Reflector: May learn best by reviewing your own experience or learning from reflecting on experiences you have had in clinical practice.
● Theorist: May prepare by reviewing the literature and reading around the subject matter of your OSCE in appropriate literature, OSCE and clinical skills books.
● Pragmatist: May learn best working alongside your mentor in clinical practice and reviewing decisions/actions you have taken in practice.

The learning style questionnaire often highlights traits of combinations of styles, e.g. pragmatist and activist, and you may be able to adapt your revision to meet both styles. For example, using this combination you may be able to learn by harnessing learning from practice and also working along-side your colleagues in your cohort in order to practise at university. It is likely that during your nursing programme you will use all four learning styles, to differing extents.

Understanding what is required

Throughout this book, each chapter will remind you to familiarize yourself with the OSCE requirements of your university as this ensures you fully understand what is expected of you (Ward and Barratt 2009). Currently there are no national nursing OSCE standards/proformas so although many universities utilize similar OSCEs the variation in requirements may vary considerably between different academic institutions.

Before commencing revision and preparation for your OSCE it is vital to understand how you will be assessed and what is assessed. Many universities' OSCE assessment strategies will be linked to education theory and commonly Bloom's (1956) taxonomy is used. Whilst this text may appear a little dated it is considered seminal work in understanding effective learning. Bloom (1956) identified a number of components to effective learning, stressing the need for education to cover all components of learning. He identified three components or domains:

1. **Cognitive domain** (knowledge),
2. **Psychomotor domain** (practical skills),
3. **Affective domain** (attitude/professional approach).

It is likely that your OSCE will test all three of these domains and you are likely to be assessed for:

1. Knowledge in relation to skill being assessed (cognitive domain),
2. Actual performance and fluency of skill (psychomotor domain),
3. Appropriate attitude and professional approach (affective domain).

A varied approach is used when testing knowledge and some universities may test knowledge at a separate station whereas others may test knowledge using a traditional written exam or online assessment/examination.

A varied approach may also be used when testing skills and some universities will test single skills, e.g. hand washing, whereas others will test this as part of a more holistic assessment, e.g. patient assessment (which also includes aspects of infection control).

Before beginning your preparation it is important that you have a clear understanding of the assessment process. It is likely that the university will have dedicated some timetabled sessions to help you prepare for the OSCE, and it is important to attend these sessions. Key questions include:

- What are the assessment criteria (it is good practice for the university to provide students with this)?
- Which skill/skills will be assessed?
- How will the skill be assessed?
- How will the knowledge be assessed?

It is vital that you have a clear understanding of the preparation required as this will enable you to plan effective preparation strategies.

Preparation for revision of knowledge underpinning your OSCE

The knowledge that is related to the OSCE you are undertaking is vitally important and you will be expected to demonstrate through observation or questioning that you understand key knowledge elements of the skill you are undertaking. It is important therefore that you revise this aspect of the OSCE.

Students may use several strategies to revise theory and it is important that you use revision strategies that suit your own learning needs. Most universities will have different resources available to ensure that all learners' needs are met. Key preparation strategies include:

- **Planning time for your revision:** You are recommended to begin reading for your OSCE at least a month before the examination. This allows you time to identify your learning requirements and knowledge deficits and to be able to fully assimilate the information before the examination date. Last minute revision is not recommended as this is likely to increase your anxiety level and detract from your performance at the OSCE.
- **Reviewing key texts:** Most universities will have adapted a key text or texts that they recommend for the course/modules. It is wise to review these texts as it is likely that they will help you to identify the knowledge that you need to learn for your OSCE and subsequent practice. Several key texts may also have an electronic database which is updated on a regular basis—it is wise to review this as well as this will be updated much more frequently and will contain more recent information.
- **Reviewing key journals:** Most academic journals frequently include updates relating to skills and knowledge and it is useful to search the university's online database for recent articles related to your OSCE. Journals tend to provide more current information than books. You will, of course, be expected to cite the most recent evidence-based practice from books and journals.
- **Reviewing key websites:** There may well be key governmental papers that you are expected to cite. It is worth viewing the National Institute for Health and Clinical Excellence (NICE) website, the Department of Health (DOH) and the Scottish Intercollegiate Guidelines Network (SIGN) websites for key papers.
- **Reviewing online university resources:** Most universities supplement text books/journals with online resources and some may have dedicated resources for the OSCE. If these are available it is essential that you review these as you will be expected to know information that is readily available.
- **Making concise notes:** It is important to note key aspects of knowledge that you can use as an aide mémoire immediately prior to the examination.

Preparation for practising the skills component of your OSCE

The actual performance and sequencing of the skill you are undertaking will be judged, usually against a set of predetermined stages (the OSCE proformas). It is vital that you are able to practise the psychomotor or skill aspects of your OSCE. It is important that you are aware of the skills criteria that you will be assessed against. This may vary between academic institutions and also may be slightly different to how you have seen a skill performed in practice.

The timing of your OSCE will influence the practising of the psychomotor component of the OSCE and different strategies will need to be adapted if your OSCE is organized before, after or during your practice placement.

Some universities may require you to undertake an OSCE before you go out into a practice area (Hart 2010). If this is the case your opportunity to practise will be limited to simulated classroom sessions. You will need to develop your psychomotor skills using the range of learning opportunities available to you at your university. These may include:

- Attending teaching sessions that prepare you to undertake the psychomotor element of the skill.
- Making effective use of any practice sessions that may be run.
- Using self-directed skills sessions as an opportunity to practise.
- Identifying any difficulties that you experience and discussing them with a member of the university's skills team or with your personal tutor.
- Reviewing university electronic resources, e.g. videos/DVDs to review key components of the skill.
- It may be useful to get together with colleagues to practice skills in the skills laboratory if you are able to organize this.
- Visiting the website www.oxfordtextbooks.co.uk to view electronic resources available alongside this book (see www.oxfordtextbooks.co.uk/orc/caballero/).
- Some universities offer virtual semi-structured assessments that guide you through the assessment of the OSCE on a computer link.

If the timing of your OSCE is during or after your practice placement then you are also able to use this opportunity to further develop your skill in the clinical area. Your clinical mentor may be able to assist you by organizing, supervising and assessing your practice (NMC 2008; Hart 2010). It is recommended that you:

- Discuss your need to adequately prepare for your OSCE with your mentor and endeavour to include elements of this in your learning contract.
- Try to observe the skill in clinical practice to enable you to build your confidence before further developing your own clinical ability.
- Try to gain clinical experience of the skill, and where appropriate seek constructive feedback from the clinical staff that will enable you to further develop your skill.
- Practise the skill as often as is appropriate. Few nurses can perfect a skill instantly and recognition of the need to take time to develop your skills is essential.

Developing the appropriate attitude and professional approach for your OSCE

A key element of the OSCE is the assessment of the affective domain. This domain is related to feelings, attitudes and caring (Quinn 2007). These can be difficult to develop, especially if you are a novice in health care, but your examiners will be looking for effective interpersonal skills and a professional approach. This is an area where many nurses struggle within an OSCE situation because they are not in a clinical area with real patients.

Many students struggle to adopt the correct approach to the 'patient' particularly if the 'patient' is a lecturer or clinical colleague. It is important that you prepare yourself by:

- Finding out who the 'patient' will be,
- Finding out if a manikin will be used.

If the patient is someone whom you know well it is important not to be overfamiliar with them in the examination. It is important that you remember that this is an examination and the normal conversations and relationships that you have with your tutor are different in an examination situation. You should endeavour (it is difficult) to treat the 'patient' as you would in clinical practice and try to demonstrate how you would effectively interact with a patient in a real clinical situation (even where a manikin is being used in the place of a patient).

Additionally your OSCE will be testing ethical aspects of the affective domain, so it is important to always seek consent from your 'patient' prior to the delivery of any clinical care. A common pitfall is to forget to gain consent and in some universities failure to gain consent will prevent a pass grade from being awarded.

If your university requires you to attend in uniform remember that your professional appearance will be judged. You should ensure that a full correct uniform is worn and strict uniform policy adhered to. This will include appropriate hairstyling and removal of jewellery, excessive make up, nail varnish and artificial nails. If you are required to attend in uniform ensure you leave sufficient time to change into your uniform at the university prior to the commencement of the OSCE. Remember to bring pens, watches and any other equipment that you will need for the OSCE with you.

Key points for preparation

- Identify your learning style and adopt a strategy that will suit you.
- Understand what is expected of you during the OSCE by discussing the examination with the academic staff that are responsible for organizing the OSCE.
- Review the key knowledge (cognitive) requirements of the skill.
- Review the key practical (psychomotor) requirements of the skill.
- Make the most of practising the skills within the university's skills laboratories.
- Take the opportunity to develop the skill in clinical practice and gain constructive feedback from your mentors.
- Ensure you prepare your correct uniform in advance.
- Psychologically prepare for the change in relationship with your examiners during the OSCE.
- Remember to gain consent and communicate effectively throughout the OSCE.
- Remember that you may be asked questions by the 'patient' and the examiner.

Box 3.1 **Remember**

- The examiners are examining for safe and effective practice; they want you to pass and for you to learn and develop from the OSCE experience.
- Effective preparation will increase your ability to pass the OSCE—reflect upon your own abilities and learn from the experience!

Table 3.1 **Revision plan**

What theory will I need to know to pass my OSCE?	How can I plan practice sessions for my OSCE?	How can I develop the right attitude and professional behaviour?

Revision plan

It may be useful to complete the revision plan in Table 3.1 and identify your own study requirements for each OSCE that you will undertake. It will be useful to develop ideas depending upon your own circumstances and learning style.

What happens after your OSCE

Once you have completed your OSCE assessment you will be informed of the outcome of the assessment. This may be on the day if it is a formative assessment or sometime afterwards if it is a summative examination that has to be processed through an examination board. You should be provided with detailed written feedback about your performance at the OSCE and it is useful to review this alongside your recollections of the experience as this will help you to learn from it. It is important that you are able to learn from the OSCE experience to enable further development of your skills and knowledge. For more information relating to learning from your OSCE please see Chapter 14.

Online resource centre

You can find further advice and revision help for your OSCEs by going online now to see **www.oxfordtextbooks.co.uk/orc/caballero/.**

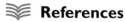 **References**

Bloom, B. (1956). *The taxonomy of educational objectives: the classification of educational goals, handbook* 1. New York: McKay.

Bloomfield, J., Pegram, A. and Jones, C. (2010). *How to pass your OSCE: a guide to success in nursing and midwifery.* Harlow: Pearson.

Hart, S. (2010). *Nursing: study and placement learning skills.* Oxford: Oxford University Press.

Honey, P. and Mumford, A. (1986). *Using your learning styles.* Maidenhead: Peter Honey.

Nursing and Midwifery Council (2008). *Standards to support learning and assessment in practice.* London: Nursing and Midwifery Council.

Quinn, F. (2007). *Principles and practice of nurse education.* Cheltenham: Nelson Thornes.

Ward, H. and Barratt, J. (2009). *Passing your advanced nursing OSCE: a guide to success in advanced clinical skills assessment.* Oxford: Radcliffe Press.

PART II
Skills

Chapter 4
Interpersonal communication
Sue Sully

 Chapter aims

This chapter will enable you to:

- Recognize the fundamental importance of effective interpersonal communication in nursing,
- Review key ideas in developing helpful interpersonal communication,
- Adapt key interpersonal skills in a variety of contexts,
- Understand how to prepare for this OSCE,
- Recognize the importance of maintaining professional boundaries.

Introduction

Nursing is an interpersonal profession (Ellis and Whittington 1981) which is to say that the majority of the goals of the profession are met through the quality and nature of relationships the nurse is able to form. Effective interpersonal communication which underpins the therapeutic relationship is a complex set of skills which require the nurse to understand the context and purpose of the interactions, in addition to being aware of their own agendas and factors which might form a barrier to effective working relationships. Historically, interpersonal communication was implicit within nursing care and by the 1980s writers such as Morrison and Burnard (1991) and Porritt (1990) had identified and explored the nature of the therapeutic relationship and interpersonal skills within nursing care. Now authors such as Stein-Parbury (2009), Burnard and Gill (2008), Maben and Griffiths (2008), Freshwater (2005) and Greenhalgh and Heath (2005) have studied and written about this area in great depth. Both the Department of Health (DOH) (2010) and the Nursing and Midwifery Council (2008) have identified the centrality of patient-led care and the nurses' ability to develop effective working relationships that enhance dignity and treat the person with compassion and care.

A therapeutic relationship is significantly different from relationships that are formed socially amongst colleagues and friends. In order to establish a relationship which is helpful it is necessary to be aware of the assumptions, expectations and feelings you carry into each new professional relationship. Without this awareness there is a real danger that your own 'noise' will make it difficult for you to be present and experience the other person as they are. In order to understand the emotional needs and concerns of the person it is necessary for you to try to understand the world of the person that you are caring for—from that person's own perspective. The nearer you can come to this the more effective will be the relationship, and the assessed needs of the patient will be more accurate and relevant. Learning about interpersonal communication within the context of nursing and the therapeutic relationship means that you will have the opportunity to develop your skills and adapt them for the purpose of caring for others.

As effective interpersonal communication can be seen as the 'bed-rock' of quality nursing care, most universities undertake this OSCE in the first year of your nursing programme. Some universities do not do a specific OSCE in this area and assess it as integral to every OSCE. You will need to check your university guidelines. The full range of interpersonal communication and developing therapeutic relationships can be assessed throughout each year of a three year undergraduate pre-registration programme with increasing degrees of complexity that reflect the complex nature of the skills involved. This chapter deals with undertaking an OSCE in the first year.

It is likely that you will be allowed between 15 and 30 minutes for this assessment and therefore you will need to have thought about the key ideas beforehand so that they can be adapted to a variety of settings both within the OSCE and in clinical practice. An OSCE is a reflection of your practice and it cannot be emphasized enough how important effective working relationships are to successful nursing care.

Key revision for your simulated examination

There are three areas that you need to focus on in order to undertake a specific interpersonal communication OSCE or if interpersonal communication is going to be assessed as part of another OSCE:

- Your interpersonal skills,
- Your own ability to relate to others,
- Your assessment of the other person.

These are assessed together and explored in the following sections.

Effective interpersonal communication

Active, sensitive listening

Hargie (2006) clearly identifies the need for effective interpersonal skills for purpose in social interactions. Firstly, active listening—this is the ability to be present for the other person and to be able to shift the focus from yourself to the other person. Active, sensitive listening is a complex skill and not one to be taken lightly as it is essential to effective working relationships with others.

Active listening is a skill that needs to be honed and the skills that an effective listener displays are to:

- Put the talker at their ease,
- Limit their own talking,
- Be attentive,
- Remove distractions,
- Show patience and do not interrupt,
- Watch for feeling words,
- Be aware of their own biases,
- Listen to paralinguistics,
- Be aware of body language,
- Use eye contact appropriately.

The phrase 'listening with a third ear' is often used to show the importance of being 'present' when listening to others. Often nurses perceive themselves as having many demands upon them and are thinking and planning ahead which means that they are only partly present for the person they are listening to. It is an art to develop the ability to be present for the other person and some of the principles that Hargie (2006) has identified are:

- Have a reason or purpose for listening,
- Suspend judgments,
- Resist distractions and fidgeting,
- Wait before responding,
- Rephrase the message accurately,
- Reflect content and search for meaning,
- Be ready to respond.

Box 4.1 shows some of the benefits of engaging in active listening which can enhance care delivery.

You may well have picked up poor listening habits and in Box 4.2 there are some points to look out for and things to avoid.

Reflecting

Geldard and Geldard (2005) see reflecting as one of the main skills involved in empathy. Simple reflection or paraphrasing is often concerned with the content of what people are saying—where the content means the 'what'. Reflection is about the feelings—the process, the 'how'. Reflecting feelings accurately depends on trying to understand how the person is feeling.

Reflecting involves both listening and trying to understand and then communicating that effort to understand. Reflecting can show that you are accepting of people.

It is not about talking down to the other person.

To reflect effectively

1. Observe facial and body movements,
2. Listen to the words and their possible meanings,
3. Tune into your own emotional reactions,
4. Sense the meaning of the communication,
5. Respond appropriately,
6. Use expressive, not stereotyped, language,

Box 4.1 **Active listening**

1. Trying to understand the person's world—what is going on for the other person.

2. Listen for total meaning. Some useful questions to ask yourself as a listener are:

   - What is this person trying to tell me?
   - What does this mean to this person?
   - How does this person see this situation?

3. Note all the cues, particularly the non-verbal and paraverbal cues, e.g.

   - Body posture
   - Eye movements
   - Hand movements
   - Inflections
   - Stressed words
   - Breathing changes
   - Facial expressions
   - Hesitancies
   - Mumbled words

4. Remember—you can only note these. Try not to make your own interpretations of them and thus seem clever. Check them out and your interpretation with the person.

   For example, a person who is hunched up in a chair, with their legs tucked under them, avoiding eye contact except to stare at you, mumbling and monosyllabic—they may be cold and tired, not angry or anxious.

> ### Box 4.2 **Active listening—what not to do**
>
> **Poor listening habits**
> 1. Not paying attention,
> 2. Pretend listening,
> 3. Listening but only hearing what you want,
> 4. Rehearsing what to say,
> 5. Interrupting the speaker in mid-sentence,
> 6. Hearing what is expected,
> 7. Feeling defensive, expecting to be attacked,
> 8. Listening for something to disagree with.
>
> **Things to avoid**
> 1. Trying to persuade people that you are right and so only hearing what you want to hear rather than what the other person might be saying.
> 2. Taking responsibility for the other person, acting like a parent. People need to be involved in decision making about their care.
> 3. Passing judgement on others, either critical or favourable. You will make judgements about others, everyone does; it is about thinking how those judgements affect your ability to work with the other person.
> 4. Platitudes and clichés show that you have not been listening to the person—this tends to be about your agenda rather than the other person.
> 5. Reassuring people, rather than listening to what is worrying and concerning them, can feel dismissive of what people are going through.

7. Ensure your vocal and bodly language agree with each other,
8. Check the accuracy of your understanding.

It could be considered pointless to actively listen to someone and for them not to know that this is occurring. The skill of simple reflecting or responding is one that is close to active listening. Other words for this type of simple reflection are paraphrasing and responding.

Simple reflection means mirroring the literal meaning of someone's words. Sometimes simple reflection is necessary; at others the skill of empathy is more appropriate where reflection of content and feeling is used.

When listening, focusing on content is usually the first step—listening to *what* the other person says. It is useful to think about the following framework when listening:

1. What—do you think you understand what they are saying?
2. Why—do you have a sense of why they are saying what they are saying?
3. Where—do you have a sense of where events took place?
4. When—do you have a sense of when things happened?
5. How—do you have a sense of how they are feeling? Angry? Happy? Sad? Frightened?

If you cannot answer these questions then further clarification may be needed. These five questions can help you to organize details and to know if the person may be leaving anything out.

You need not respond by repetition or parroting what the other person said but by paraphrasing in your own words, which captures the main points in a brief statement and thus checks out your understanding with the other person.

Examples of this may be (although you will probably use your own similar phrases):

'It sounds like......'

'So you are saying that.....'

'In other words......'

Paraphrasing, responding or simple reflection are all the terms that are used to discuss the reflection of content and are considered the first stage in skills development for an empathic response.

Questioning

Hargie (2006) and Stein-Parbury (2009) recognize the importance of questions as tools to obtain information. They can be overused by nurses who often feel under pressure and that they have little time and therefore ask questions as a way of gaining information quickly. This is not always helpful because information gets missed and it means that there is a shift of focus away from the other person back to the nurse.

The following can be helpful:

1. Use open questions. This allows the person to choose the direction that the conversation will take. If the person has something that they want to 'get off their chests' it can be infuriating if the nurse is constantly steering the conversation away; constantly asking questions is one of the most effective ways of preventing effective interpersonal communication.
2. Wrongly used, questions can create an expectation that nurses will provide solutions to other people's problems. The emphasis is on using questions as aids to problem solving.
3. Are there so many questions that it seems like an interrogation?
4. Who are you asking the question for?
   Is it idle curiosity?
   Is it to gain information?
   Is it to avoid an uncomfortable subject?
   Is it to lead the person in the direction that you want to go?

Open questions can help to:

- Seek clarification,
- Encourage exploration,
- Establish understanding,
- Gauge feelings,
- Establish some clarification.

Things to avoid:

- Closed questions—unless you want to elicit information or establish facts,
- Curiosity questions,
- Questions which begin with 'is', 'are', 'do', 'did',
- Too many questions that give the impression of an interrogation,
- Questions which put the words into people's mouths,
- Probing questions which the other person is not yet ready to answer,
- Poorly timed questions that interrupt and hinder the other person's conversation.

Clarifing and summarizing

Clarifying and summarizing are two interpersonal skills that are linked to listening and questioning. They help to show the person who is talking that the nurse is trying to listen and understand what is being said.

Clarifying shows the other person what you are struggling to understand as you check out your understanding of what is being said. Here are some handy thoughts:

1. If you are not sure what the person means by what they are saying, it is important to get them to explain further to avoid confusion.
2. Again this helps to confirm to the person that you are actually listening and interested in what they have to say (provided you are not doing it too often).
3. If you do not clarify statements you are unsure of, there is a chance that you will respond inappropriately, or ask questions that the other person feels they have already explained. In this case the person may be justifiably angry and lose confidence in your relationship.
4. An important part of clarification is listening to the client's feedback and then making adjustments accordingly.
5. Clarification is particularly useful in developing empathy.
6. Effective clarification provides a model on which clients may model their communication.

Summarizing can indicate what you have understood from what the other person was saying and can include both what is said and how it is said. It does not mean that you have to accurately repeat everything that has been said but is about trying to convey your understanding. Most people do not actually listen to what they are saying and having a summary repeated to them can also help them to clarify what the issues might be for them.

1. It allows you to tie up all the pieces that you have heard so far before going any further.
2. It shows the person that you are paying attention to what they are saying and reinforces your commitment to listening (it may also show the person that you are not listening and gives them the opportunity to put you straight).
3. It allows the person to hear repeated to them what they have said, probably in a more concise way. This can be extremely valuable.
4. When people are distressed they can seldom see the aspects of their difficulties clearly. To hear the problems clearly stated can often put things into focus and help the person realize that the problems are not as overwhelming as they had thought.
5. Summarizing allows for a break and a review. It creates space and can slow things down.
6. It provides a basis to plan care.
7. It helps you when feeling stuck.
8. It helps people to view their problems from a different perspective.

Box 4.3 Interpersonal skills self-assessment sheet (adapted from work by Sarah Brown)

Name: Date:

Evaluate yourself and your interpersonal skills in the following ways by ticking in the boxes.

A Already do this effectively.   ☐
B Do this, but need to work on it to be more effective.   ☐
C A new concept to think about/learn to use.   ☐
D Find this difficult to use/apply.   ☐

	Interpersonal skills	A	B	C	D
1	Able to listen actively and remember.				
2	Able to reflect feelings.				
3	Able to summarize what the other person has said.				
4	Able to clarify when I do not understand.				
5	Can use skills appropriately.				
6	Am in touch with own inner world and feelings.				
7	Can create a safe relationship.				
8	Am aware of my impact on others.				
9	Can empathize with another's feelings and communicate this understanding.				
10	Am able to be present in the moment.				
11	My non-verbal behaviour shows that I am able to listen.				

Attitudes

1. How much respect and acceptance of others do I feel? How do I know I communicate these attitudes?
2. Am I at one with myself, and how do I know I communicate this genuineness?
3. Which judgmental attitudes that could make listening to others difficult am I aware of having, and how will I deal with them?
4. What are my strengths as a person using interpersonal skills, and what skills do I use well now?
5. What are my limitations as a person using interpersonal skills, and what skills do I need to learn/improve?
6. What stops me giving people my full attention?
7. What can I do so that I can give people my full attention?

Action

List two areas that you hope to change and for each area identify two ways in which you will know that you have changed.

1. I would like to change/improve ....
   I will know that I have achieved this by:
   (a)
   (b)
2. I would like to change/improve ....
   I will know that I have achieved this by:
   (a)
   (b)

Utilizing these approaches in your OSCE examination

At this station it is likely that you will be given an outline of a scenario setting the scene and a written scenario before being asked to meet the person you are to work with. Some universities may use 'actors' or members of staff for this station and you will need to check the guidelines for your course. In some universities they do not specifically assess this element of nursing care and instead include as part of every OSCE and again you will need to check the guidelines for your course. This can be a formative or a summative assessment of your abilities and the aim is to provide a relatively safe environment to explore your abilities and recognize what you do well as well as areas that you might want to develop during your education programme. You will be assessed on:

1. Your ability to use interpersonal skills appropriately and for purpose,
2. Your ability to recognize your own processes and how you might be influencing the situation,
3. Your ability to work with the person,
4. Your recognition of the impact of verbal and non-verbal skills,
5. Your professional attitude,
6. Dignity and respect shown to the person,
7. Ability to report back your findings and assessment of the situation.

It can be helpful to do a self-assessment of your interpersonal skills in preparation for the assessment. Remember to be as honest as you can and also not to be too hard on yourself. It can help to think what someone who knows you might say in filling in the questions.

You will be given the time constraints for the OSCE and you need to be aware of timing the interaction and remember not to go over the time. Examples of OSCEs are in Boxes 4.4 and 4.5.

Example of an interpersonal communication OSCE

Box 4.4 **Written scenario**

You are working on a stroke rehabilitation ward for four weeks and on this day have been asked to look after Mr Birch. You have not looked after Mr Birch before as you have been working in other parts of the ward.

The patient

Mr Geoffrey Birch is a 76 year old retired bank manager who was admitted with a stroke and left sided hemiparesis.

He had worked as a bank manager in the local town for 25 years and retired 11 years ago. He nursed his wife who had had breast cancer for 5 years and who died 3 years ago. They have no children and he has one sister who has lived in South Africa for 50 years. He has no other living relatives.

Until his stroke he had played golf 3–4 times a week and is a member of the local Masonic lodge.

He is trying to decide whether to go home to his large detached house with a substantial garden which his wife used to look after or to go into a warden controlled flat.

In handover, the nurse in charge asked if you would talk with Mr Birch about his decision as it seems he is finding it difficult to decide what to do.

Step by step guide

Setting up an effective working relationship with a person you are nursing starts from the moment that you and the patient can see each other as you will start to make decisions about how they might be feeling, what they might be thinking and your response to them and, of course, they will be doing the same. This is an interaction with purpose and that will influence what you do and how you do it. This means the other person has an issue and you have been asked to explore this with them. It may be that Mr Birch will not reach a decision when talking with you; however, the aim is to help him in that decision making process. Be aware of barriers to effective interpersonal communication such as deafness or noise in the environment.

Remember that you will need to decontaminate your hands before approaching the person.

Introduction

It can help to acknowledge the person with either a nod or a smile before you decontaminate your hands. When you approach the person, greet them and introduce yourself, who you are and why you are there. Ask the person how they would like to be addressed.

Find a place to sit near them, drawing up a chair if necessary, face them and do not stand over them.

Remember that the interaction is time limited and you need to think about ending as you start.

Active listening and being present are essential in developing effective working relationships with people.

It can be useful once you have introduced yourself to ask an open question.

'I have 15 minutes and I was wondering how you are feeling today.'

Or an alternative could be to summarize what you know.

'I have 20 minutes with you now, and I understand that you are thinking about moving and maybe living in a warden controlled flat. I would imagine that is a hard decision for you to make.'

Quick summary

1. The interaction starts from the moment you see each other,
2. Decontaminate your hands,
3. Introduce yourself,
4. Ask what the person would like to be called,
5. Sit facing them,
6. Tell the person how long you have with them.

Moving forward

Whilst the conversation needs to be led by the other person (a reflection of patient centred care) you have a reason for being there as well and it can be hard at times to manage the balance between these two. You have been asked to talk to him about making a decision so that is your 'agenda' and this might not be the same for Mr Birch. It is important to respond to the person and what they want to talk about and also remember that you want to talk about his decision to move.

Do not talk over the other person or interrupt them with words. Let them finish what they are saying or if you feel that you need to say something, then give a non-verbal cue such as leaning forward, using a facial expression, or when they take a breath then say:

'I just wanted to say something, if that is OK...'

Your non-verbal communication is important as it can convey that you are listening to what is being said and nodding in response can be helpful, although avoid looking like a 'nodding-dog'. Para-verbal responses such as 'hrm' can also be used sparingly. Check out what you might be conveying:

1. Are you fidgeting?
2. Is your mind wandering?
3. Are you rushing?

It can be helpful to take a deep breath and bring your attention back to Mr Birch. Remember to do this 'check out' on yourself regularly during the OSCE.

Think about Mr Birch's non-verbal cues as well, e.g.

- His breathing,
- Facial expressions,
- His eye movements,
- Sentences left unfinished,
- Words that are stressed,
- Hand movements.

All of these can you help you try to understand what is going on for Mr Birch and give you some indication of how he might be feeling, as well as his thought processes. You can only note these behaviours and think about what they might mean. *You do not know* what they mean, only what you think they mean.

Keep the balance towards reflection rather than questioning. If asking questions think about why you are asking them—is it to help the other person understand or idle curiosity?

Clarifying your understanding can be more helpful than asking questions.

'So, if I understand what you are saying, Mr Birch, you would like to give up your house because it is too big for you now and you cannot manage the garden; however, you are worried and sad because it was the house that you and your wife lived in together for such a long time and it has memories of her.'

Remember it is not just what the other person is saying, but also about their emotions and you need to acknowledge those as well.

It is not about agreeing with what Mr Birch says, it is about:

1. Helping him to explore the options that he thinks that he might have,
2. Responding to questions that he might have,
3. Recognizing the limits of your knowledge and finding out the appropriate information for him and letting him know,
4. You being able to give an account to the nurse in charge of what Mr Birch said and having a plan to help him to decide.

Quick summary

1. Actively listen,
2. Be present for the other person,
3. On balance it is more about them than you,
4. Be aware of your body language and that of the other person,
5. Ask questions sparingly,
6. On balance, reflect and clarify more than ask questions,
7. Be led by the other person and remember you have a reason for being there,
8. The interaction is time limited.

Ending

Keep an eye on the time and when there is about 2–3 minutes left, tell Mr Birch that you are coming to the end of time. It might be helpful to say something like:

'Mr Birch, I have just noticed that we have about 3 minutes left and I thought it might be helpful if I summarize what I think we have talked about.'

Remember a summary can help the other person as well as you. People do not always listen to what they say and having someone summarize that can be useful and can help to clarify points and could help Mr Birch think about the way forward. It can be a way of showing that you were listening to Mr Birch and he can correct any misunderstandings or inaccuracies which are inevitable when you listen and make sense of the other person's story. It is also a way for you to acknowledge some of the difficulties that Mr Birch might be facing and a way forward to deal with those. It can be the basis for a plan.

'This seems like a really difficult decision for you. You know that you have a weakness in your right leg and arm that means that managing at home will be very difficult for you because it is such a large house and garden. However, this is your home and was your home with your wife. She died there and that makes leaving very hard. These are not easy decisions to make. You seem to be nearer to making a decision to move into a warden controlled flat and you know that you have until the end of the week to make the final decision. However, you are finding the time pressure hard as well. I have agreed to chat with your named nurse and tell her where you are in terms of making a decision today and that it might be useful for you to go and see the warden controlled flat. I will speak to the occupational therapist about arranging a visit and also for her to come and see you today when she visits the ward. I will be with her so that we can all talk together. I appreciate you being so honest with me, thank you.'

Quick summary

1. Let the person know when there are about 2–3 minutes left,
2. Offer a summary or let them summarize and you add what you think is important when appropriate,
3. Include *what* the person has said and also *how* they might be feeling (angry, happy, sad or frightened),
4. Be tentative in the summary because you may be wrong,
5. It is a collaboration so be prepared to be corrected,
6. Tell the person you will be talking to other relevant people about what you have discussed,
7. Say what you think you have agreed,
8. State what the plan is,
9. Thank them.

When you have finished the interaction with the person, you may need to report back to the examiner as though they were the nurse in charge although this is not always the case and you will need to check the university guidelines. When reporting back then you need to be:

1. Clear,
2. Concise,
3. Give the highlights that are relevant in a professional manner,
4. At this point you are the patient's representative,
5. Say what the plan is and the way forward.

So an example might be:

'Hello, I have chatted with Mr Birch and he is closer to making a decision about moving. He has moved towards living in the warden controlled flat however he has not finally decided. He is finding it a hard decision to make and although he is finding it hard he knows he has to decide by the end of the week. I know the occupational therapist is on the ward today and he would like to talk to her about arranging a visit and I have said that I will be with him when he chats to her. If it works out would it be OK for me to go on the visit to the flat as well?'

If your interpersonal communication is to be assessed as part of another OSCE, e.g. clinical skills, then there are some additional things that you can think about.

Example of interpersonal communication within a clinical skills OSCE

Step by step guide

All effective nursing care is based on a working relationship between the nurse and the person and therefore it could be that in your university they do not assess interpersonal communication directly in an OSCE but as an integral part of what is being assessed (see OSCE example box 4.5). It can be helpful to complete the self-evaluation form from earlier in the chapter as a way of preparing yourself for this element (see Table 4.1). The three areas identified here are a useful guide:

1. Introduction,
2. Moving forward,
3. Ending.

Box 4.5 **Written scenario**

You are asked to undertake physical parameter observations and recordings of blood pressure, temperature, respirations, pulse and oxygen saturation in the OSCE room and your interpersonal communication will be assessed as part of this OSCE.

The patient

Miss Mary Pierce was admitted during the afternoon with abdominal pain following a period of 4 months of seeing her General Practitioner (GP) for investigations. During that time her abdominal pain had become more intense and her abdomen had become distended. Her dress size has gone from a size 10 to a size 14 to accommodate her increased girth measurement. She has lived in the same house that she was born in and had worked in the local primary school as a teacher until she retired 10 years previously.

Whilst you are undertaking and recording the data that you have gathered, Miss Pierce says that she is scared as she has not been in hospital before although she visited on numerous occasions when her mother and father had been in the same hospital. In fact her mother had died in the same ward five years ago. Her mother had died of liver cancer when she was 93 years old and although Miss Pierce is not the same age she is worried.

Setting up an effective working relationship with a person you are nursing starts from the moment that you and the patient see each other as you will start to make decisions about how they might be feeling, what they might be thinking and your response to them and, of course, they will be doing the same.

Introduction

After you have decontaminated your hands, greet Miss Pierce and introduce yourself and ask permission to undertake the observations. Ask her how she would like to be addressed, e.g.

> 'Hello Miss Pierce, I am student nurse .... I need to record your blood pressure, temperature, pulse and respirations if that is OK? I am not sure what to call you. Do you prefer Miss Pierce or Mary?'

Be aware of standing next to rather than 'over' Miss Pierce.

Quick summary

1. Introduce yourself,
2. Say why you are there,
3. Ask how the person would prefer to be addressed,
4. Be aware of standing *next to* rather than *over* the person.

As stated Miss Pierce engages you in conversation and you will need to respond to her as well as carry out the recordings that you have been assigned to undertake. The difficulty will be the balance between listening and engaging with what is being said and doing the tasks.

Moving forward

Depending on the timing of the station you need to decide if you will respond to what is being said directly or whether you will carry out the assigned tasks and let Miss Pierce know that you have heard what she has said and arrange to come back. If the timing of the station is short as it is likely to be, then acknowledging what has been said and arranging to come back may be the most appropriate option. This recognizes the patient-led nature of care and also that you have a purpose for being with the person that also needs to be taken into account.

Active, sensitive listening is necessary and recognizing that Miss Pierce says that she is scared about two things—that she might have cancer and that her mother died in the same ward that she is in now.

Remember that this is about listening to **what** is said and also about **how** the person seems to be emotionally and responding to both elements. You will need to be aware of Miss Pierce's non-verbal communication as well as what words she is using. You will also need to be aware of your own response to what is said.

Remember that reassuring is not appropriate (as it disregards people's concerns and their importance) and that acknowledgement is reassuring. So you may say something such as:

> 'That sounds really horrible for you, Miss Pierce, to be in the same ward as where your mother died. I would imagine that it brings back memories.'

> 'I would imagine that this is a scary time for you—not knowing what is going on and having to come into hospital for investigations and then find yourself on the same ward as where your mother died.'

The focus of the station needs to be addressed and you need to also think about why Miss Pierce has told you, rather than another team member, and told you when she did. Often people worry that others will think them 'silly' or they are dismissive of what they are feeling and it is important that you acknowledge in your own words what is said and make a plan for coming back if appropriate. You will need to communicate the information you have gained to the relevant person on the ward, either the named nurse or the nurse in charge.

Quick summary

1. Acknowledge *what* is said and *how* the person seems to be feeling,
2. Avoid the use of questions,
3. Do not reassure them that everything will be OK,
4. Draw on the skill of reflection,
5. Be aware of your own response to what is said.

Ending

Complete the task at hand and then summarize for Miss Pierce what you have heard and if appropriate make a plan with her. So you may say something like:

> 'I have to record your blood pressure, etc., Miss Pierce, and then I need to go. I wish I could stay a little longer because this seems a difficult and frightening time for you. However, I can come back later and we can have a chat if that suits you?'

It is alright to leave as not all difficult issues have to be dealt with immediately. However, it is important to let the person know that you have heard what they have said and how they might be feeling as this shows respect and compassion for what the person is going through. You are not responsible for how they feel but you are responsible for how you react to the situation.

Quick summary

1. Recognize that you are there for a purpose,
2. Not all difficulties have to be addressed straight away,
3. You *are not* responsible for how someone feels,
4. You *are* responsible for what you do in response to the situation,
5. It is OK to come back if the person wants you to,
6. Either report the information to the examiner or state that you would report the information to the nurse in charge, whichever is appropriate within the context of the station.

Examiners' marking criteria

Table 4.1 **Example of examiners' marking criteria**

Student's name and cohort year	
Expected performance criteria	Demonstrated Yes/No
Decontaminates their hands before approaching the person.	
Introduces themselves.	
Asks what to call the person.	
Sits or stands facing person and does not loom.	

Table 4.1 (*continued*)

Student's name and cohort year	
Expected performance criteria	Demonstrated Yes/No
Appears aware of any barriers to interpersonal communication such as physical barriers or noise.	
Signs of active listening.	
Reflecting skills—acknowledges what is said.	
Reflecting skills—acknowledges what the person might be feel.	
Clarifying.	
Summarizing.	
Appropriate use of open questions.	
Appropriate use of closed questions.	
Professional approach.	
Being present.	
States time limit of interaction.	
States a way forward in negotiation with the person.	
Does not interrupt inappropriately.	
Does not talk over the other person.	
Picks up on non-verbal cues of other person.	
Reports back to examiner (nurse in charge) in a factual, clear and concise manner.	

Examiners' questions

Questions that the examiner might ask will be related to your performance. Examples are provided in Box 4.6.

Box 4.6 **Example of examiners' questions**

1. What was the most important moment for you in this interaction?
2. How did you feel during the interaction and how did this impact on your ability to relate to the other person?

General questions might include:

1. What makes interpersonal communication effective?
2. Why is it important to try to develop effective nurse–patient/client relationships?
3. How might effective nurse–patient/client relationships be established?

See the end of the chapter for answers.

✗ Common errors at this station

Some of the common errors at this station are a failure to:

- Decontaminate your hands,
- Greet the other person,
- Introduce yourself,
- Ask what the other person likes to be called,
- Be aware of non-verbal cues,
- Be aware of your own responses to the other person,
- Actively listen,
- Recognize that you are there for a purpose,
- Offer patient-led care,
- Have a plan that is negotiated with the other person for a way forward if appropriate,
- Keep good timing,
- Report clearly and concisely.

➕ Top tips for passing this station

Try to avoid the common errors and also think about the following:

- Always speak in the first person when referring to yourself—so '*I understand that you are...*'
- Use the word 'and' instead of 'but'—but often sounds like a prelude to criticism.
- Take a deep breath before you think—OSCEs can be stressful and you can forget to breathe into the base of your lungs and you need oxygen to think.
- Think before you speak—although time at the station can be short, do not rush—develop a measured pace.
- Do not ask too many questions—remember the other useful skills such as reflecting, clarifying and summarizing.
- Do not fidget.
- Do not concentrate on paperwork rather than the other person—people are important.

≋ References

Burnard, P. and Gill, P. (2008). *Culture, Communication and Nursing: A Multicultural Guide.* Harlow: Pearson Education.

Department of Health (2010). *Front Line Care: the future of nursing and midwifery in England. Report of the Prime Minister's Commission on the Future of Nursing and Midwifery in England 2010.* London: Department of Health, Her Majesty's Stationery Office.

Ellis, R. and Whittington, D. (1981). *Guide to Social Skills Training.* London: Croom and Helm.

Freshwater, D. (2005). *Counselling Skills for Nurses, Midwives and Health Visitors.* Oxford: Oxford University Press.

Geldard, K. and Geldard, D. (2005). Practical *Counselling Skills Training: An Integrative Approach.* London: Palgrave Macmillan.

Greenhalgh, T. and Heath, I. (2005). *Measuring Quality in the Therapeutic Relationship.* London: Kings Fund.

Hargie, O.D.W. (ed.) (2006). *Handbook of Communication Skills.* London: Routledge.

Maben, J. and Griffiths, P. (2008). *Nurses in Society: Starting the Debate.* London: Nursing Research Unit, King's College London.

Morrison, P. and Burnard, P. (1991). *Caring and Communicating: Interpersonal Relationship in Nursing.* London: Palgrave Macmillan.

Nursing and Midwifery Council (2008). *Code of Conduct for Nursing and Midwifery.* London: Nursing and Midwifery Council.

Porritt, L. (1990). *Interaction Strategies: An Introduction for Health Professionals* (2nd edn). London: Churchill Livingstone.

Stein-Parbury, J. (2009). *Patient and Person: Interpersonal Skills in Nursing* (4th edn). London: Churchill Livingstone.

Appendix: answers to examiners' questions

Answers to general questions might include:

1. What makes interpersonal communication effective? Think about the following for example:
   * My ability to actively listen to the other person
   * My ability to try to understand the other person
   * My ability to use interpersonal skills effectively such as reflecting, summarizing and clarifying
   * That the other person feels that they have been heard and taken seriously
   * My ability to attend to the patient's emotional needs
   * My ability to convey complex information in a way that is understood

2. Why is it important to try to develop effective nurse–patient/client relationships? Think about the following for example:
   * Because nursing care relies on effective working relationships with patients
   * Because nurses work with people
   * Because effective working relationships are the bedrock to nursing care
   * Because the patient matters

3. How might effective nurse–patient/client relationships be established? Think about the following for example:
   * By the nurse being aware of how they are and how others might see them
   * By the nurse being able to attentively listen
   * By the nurse using questions sparingly and with purpose
   * By the nurse drawing on other interpersonal skills such as reflecting when appropriate
   * By the nurse attending to the content and process of the interaction
   * By the nurse being able to convey complex information in a way that can be understood

Chapter 5
Hand hygiene and infection control

Jane Lovegrove

Chapter aims

This chapter will provide an overview of hand hygiene and infection control. This will enable you to:

- Understand why this important skill is assessed using OSCE,
- Revise key material in relation to this skill,
- Follow a step by step guide to effective hand washing,
- Understand how to prepare and revise for this OSCE,
- Highlight common problems at this station and identify how these may be avoided.

Introduction

Each year hundreds of millions of people contract an infection while in the receipt of heath care. At any time 1.4 million people worldwide are suffering from an infectious complication associated with health care (WHO 2005). **Health care acquired infections** not only lead to pain discomfort, disability, and possible death for the recipient but also place a huge emotional and physical burden on relatives and carers. In England and Wales an average of one in 11,000 people die of a hospital acquired infection (HAI) each year; this figure rises to 1 in 300 for patients over the age of 80 (Bandolier 2006). Hospital admission is now a major risk factor for health care related infection (Gould 2009). In 2007 around 9,000 people in England died with an MRSA bloodstream infection or related *Clostridium difficile* infection (National Audit Office 2009). These figures do not include deaths from other HAIs so in fact the number of deaths from HAIs could be greater. In addition, it is also believed that many people die from a health care acquired infection which is not identified on the death certificate. In England, health care related infections have been estimated to cost a billion pounds annually (WHO 2005).

The World Health Organization has identified hand hygiene as the primary measure to reduce infections (WHO 2009). Everyone involved in the provision of health care must be trained in effective hand decontamination (NICE 2003). Unclean hands move microorganisms from one place to another. Transmission of infection by hands has been identified with recent hospital outbreaks of MRSA and *Clostridium difficile*. Good hand hygiene is one of the most effective methods of reducing hospital acquired infections. Hand decontamination removes transient bacteria acquired from recent contact with an infected item or person. While hand decontamination is advocated before contact with every patient regardless of setting, patients in hospital are at greatest risk of acquiring an infection. In the UK 7.6% of patients admitted to hospital become infected. In England the figure is even higher at 8.19% (Nazarko 2008).

It is essential for health care students to not only be able to perform effective hand washing, but also understand the principles of the procedure, as well as the possible physical, emotional and financial consequences of failing to perform hand hygiene.

Key revision for your simulated examination

While the evidence that the simple act of hand washing reduces infection and saves lives has been known for a long time, compliance among health care workers remains an issue throughout the world (WHO 2005). Health care staff continue to fail to wash their hands with the result that thousands of patients in England and Wales die each year of an infection acquired in hospital (Nazarko 2008).

Microorganisms on the hands

Microorganisms cannot be seen by the naked eye. The term microorganisms includes bacteria, viruses and some fungi. Typically there are between 10,000 and 10 million bacteria on each hand (HPA 2011). The skin forms a protective layer which prevents these microorganisms from entering the body. However, if the skin integrity is breached, bacteria that are harmless on the outside of the skin may enter the deeper tissues of the body and cause infection. Some of these bacteria are found on the skin at all times and these are termed 'resident bacteria'. Resident bacteria live permanently in hair follicles and sebaceous glands (Horton 1999). Other bacteria are picked up and carried by a person for a limited period of time; these are termed 'transient bacteria'. Transient bacteria are acquired by contact with another person or object (Parker 1999) and are found on the surface of the skin in the stratum corneum (WHO 2009). *Escherichia coli, Staphylococcus aureus* and *Pseudomonas* are examples of transient bacteria that may be found on the skin. During the 1970s, research found that infections found in patients were frequently caused by the same strains of bacteria found on health workers' hands (Gould 2009). The majority of transient bacteria may be physically removed by hand washing or killed by bactericidal solutions such as alcohol rubs. The purpose of hand hygiene is to remove dirt and reduce the number of bacteria on the hands.

When hand hygiene should be performed

To assist health care workers conceptualize the risk of infection, the WHO (2009) divides the health care setting into the **patient zone** and the **health care area.** The patient zone contains the patient and his/her immediate surroundings, for example the bed, linen, locker, bed table, call bell, etc. It also contains all equipment touched by health care workers when in the vicinity of the patient, that is infusion pumps, intravenous infusions, oxygen flow meters, monitors, etc. The health care area contains all surfaces outside the patient zone, which should be viewed as being covered in microorganisms potentially harmful to the patient.

In 2006 the WHO identified the following five key moments for hand hygiene in health care contexts:

- **Before patient contact:** To reduce the risk of exogenous infection, hand hygiene should be performed after last contact with an object outside the patient zone and before the first contact within the patient zone, for example after closing the curtains and before moving the patient's bed table.
- **Before an aseptic task:** Once in the patient zone there is a risk of endogenous infection by the transfer of microorganisms from a surface or skin to an open wound or **intravenous**

infusion site, for example if a health care worker moves the bed table and then proceeds to touch an intravenous infusion site.

- **After exposure or risk of exposure to body fluid** (and after glove removal): After contact with body fluid or any site where there may be body fluids hand hygiene should be performed. This reduces the risk of transmission of microorganisms from a 'colonized' site to a clean site. Gloves are used by health care workers as a 'second skin', but they are not a sufficient barrier and hand hygiene needs to be performed after glove removal.

- **After patient contact, i.e. after touching a patient:** When a health care worker moves out of the patient zone, there is a risk of transmission of microorganisms from the patient to the health care area. To prevent this, the health care worker should clean their hands after the final contact with the patient.

- **After contact with patient surroundings:** After touching any object or furniture in the patient's immediate surroundings, even without touching the patient, hand hygiene should be performed, for example a health care worker may move one patient's chair in order to access another patient. This also raises the issue that all objects taken from a patient zone should be destroyed, or cleaned prior to being used for a second patient.

How hand hygiene can be performed

If hands are not soiled the use of an alcohol based solution is preferred. The WHO has identified the following situations when hands should be washed as opposed to cleaned using alcohol rub (WHO 2005).

Hands should be washed with soap and water when:

- Visibly dirty,
- Contaminated with proteinaceous material,
- Visibly soiled with blood or any other body fluid,
- Where exposure to spore forming bacteria is suspected or evident,
- Following urination or defecation.

Hand washing with soap and water

Water alone is not suitable or acceptable as water will not remove substances such as fats and oils (WHO 2009). Hand washing with plain soap and water will physically remove microorganisms and prevent them being transferred to a patient or inanimate object, but does not kill bacteria. Hand washing with soap and water is acceptable in low risk situations such as blowing the nose and visiting the lavatory in the home. This is called a social hand wash (Horton 1999). In this situation liquid soap is preferable to bars of soap as bars of soap are difficult to dry and may crack providing space for bacteria to reside. Patients in a hospital environment should be encouraged to use liquid soap. However, if patients insist on using bars of soap, the bar should be rinsed after use and stored in a manner that allows the bar to dry between use. Disposable liquid soap dispensers are preferable and refilling of soap dispensers discouraged.

Antiseptic handwashing

Antiseptic agents such as chlorhexidine gluconate or povidone iodine have bactericidal action. Chlorhexidene gluconate continues to kill bacteria after being applied, but is more effective against gram positive bacteria than gram negative bacteria, tubercle bacteria, fungi and viruses. Iodo-phores, solutions that contain iodine, have a wide range of action and are effective against both gram negative and gram positive bacteria, tubercle bacillus, fungi and viruses (Horton 1999). An antiseptic agent should be used prior to invasive procedures such as aseptic technique and urinary catheterization (Gould 2009). Antiseptic solution is also advocated where patients are vulnerable, i.e. those with low resistance to infection, the new born, those in intensive care and patients who are immunosuppressed.

Bare below the elbow, rings, wrist watches and nails

In 2007 in an attempt to clarify uniform policy, the Department of Health issued guidelines for developing policies for uniforms and work wear (DOH 2007). The guidelines state that short sleeved clothing should be worn as cuffs have been found to become heavily contaminated with bacteria and are more likely to come into contact with patients. Wrist watches and jewellery harbour infection as do long and false nails and therefore should not be worn. Nails should be no longer than 0.5 cm (WHO 2005). Skin under rings has been shown to be more heavily colonized with microorganisms than skin on fingers without rings (WHO 2009). Rings with sharp surfaces are not acceptable in any health care setting as they are more likely to harbour microorganisms, may puncture gloves and present a risk of scratching a patient. A smooth plain ring may be acceptable if it can be moved and the finger washed beneath; however, even these are not acceptable in high risk situations such as an operating theatre (WHO 2009). While these guideline are primarily targeted at staff who have direct contact with patients, they are also advocated for non-clinical staff (DOH 2007).

Hand hygiene using soap/antiseptic solution and water

When washing with soap or an antiseptic solution and water the following actions are advocated by the National Patient Safety Agency (NPSA 2007):

- Wet hands,
- Apply sufficient soap to cover all surfaces of the hands,
- Rub hands palm to palm,
- Rub back of each hand with the palm of the other hand with fingers interlaced,
- Rub palm to palm with fingers interlaced,
- Rub backs of fingers with opposing palms,
- Rub each thumb clasped in opposite hand using rotational movement,
- Rub tips of fingers in opposite palm in a circular motion,
- Rub each wrist with opposite hand,
- Rinse hands under running water,
- Take care not to contaminate hands on the tap or sink,
- Prevent contamination by using elbows to turn off taps,
- Dry thoroughly with a single use towel.

This procedure should take 40–60 seconds.

Drying

Drying of hands is important as damp hands spread 1,000 times more microbes than dry hands (HPA 2011). Cloth towels are not advocated for the health care setting as they are difficult to dry between use and damp environments increase the risk of bacterial growth. Cloth towels may increase the risk of cross infection when used repeatedly or by more than one person. If cloth towels are used repeatedly, e.g. in a patient's home, they should be thoroughly dried between use and ideally changed daily (Parker 1999).

Hot air dryers are effective if hands are held under the dryer until dry, but this takes longer than drying hands using towels, so they are not advocated for use in clinical areas, where hands need to be dried quickly. In addition hand dryers are very noisy and may disturb patients, particularly at night.

Absorbent paper towels dry the hands quickly and effectively. Hands should be dried from fingers to wrists and the towel discarded to avoid recontamination from skin above the wrist that has not been washed. Foot operated bins are required to avoid the need to touch the bin with the hand. Paper towels should be soft to encourage use and avoid damage to the skin that may result from frequent hand drying using harder more abrasive towels. Patting the hands dry has also been advocated as a means of reducing the risk of abrasion (WHO 2009).

Studies comparing the efficacy of hand dryers versus paper towels have been found to be inconclusive. Further studies are required.

Hand hygiene using alcohol hand rub

Hand rubs should only be used on hands that are physically clean (WHO 2005). Alcohol hand rubs usually contain both alcohol and a bactericidal agent. Alcohol kills bacteria more effectively than other agents but needs to dry before full effect is obtained (Horton 1999). Alcohol solutions containing 60–80% alcohol are the most effective; however, although alcohol has a rapid action it has negligible residual bactericidal effect. For this reason alcohol solutions are normally combined with an antiseptic agent for prolonged activity against **pathogens** (WHO 2009).

When using alcohol hand rubs, the hands should be dry before application. A small amount of hand rub sufficient to cover all surfaces of the hands should be applied to a cupped hand. Having applied the alcohol rub, the same actions to those advocated for a soap and water hand wash should be performed until the hands are dry. The more gel applied the longer the hand rub is required. Once the hands are dry they are safe and ready for use. The advocated time taken for hand hygiene using alcohol hand rub is 20–30 seconds (NPSA 2007).

Alcohol kills many different types of bacteria, including MRSA (Gould 2009). It also has a high capacity to kill viruses such as the flu virus, the common cold and HIV although it is not effective against Novovirus. In addition endospores of some bacteria such as *Clostridium difficile* are relatively resistant to alcohol hand rubs.

The NPSA and WHO advocate the use of alcohol rubs in health care settings as they are quick to use and may be placed wherever there is a need to perform hand hygiene (NPSA 2007; WHO 2009). This facilitates compliance as staff are more likely to clean their hands if the means of doing so is immediately available. In addition some studies have shown that the use of alcohol based hand rubs is more effective in reducing the risk of pathogen transmission than soap and water (WHO 2009).

Skin care

Health care workers who have hand dermatitis have been found to colonize bacteria for prolonged periods of time (WHO 2009). It is therefore essential that the skin on health workers, hands is intact and in good condition. Hand lotions should be used to keep skin in good condition but should only be provided in dispensers to avoid the risk of contamination.

Use of gloves

The use of gloves does not replace the need for hand hygiene. Hands should be cleansed prior to the use of gloves using the criteria in 'Hand hygiene using soap/antiseptic solution and water'. Gloves should be worn when there is contact or risk of contact with any body fluid, mucous membranes or non-intact skin. Gloves may also be worn to reduce the risk of transmission of germs from one person to another or to reduce the risk of hands being contaminated from a contaminated surface as hand washing may not remove all pathogens. Gloves should be removed immediately after use and should not be worn for the care of more than one patient or for contact with more than one body site of a patient (WHO 2005). Hand hygiene also needs to be performed after removal of gloves as gloves may become inadvertently punctured. In addition hands sweat while gloves are being worn causing bacteria to move from areas under the nails and deeper layers of skin thus increasing the number of bacteria on the surface of the skin (Burd 2006). It is also possible that hands may be contaminated with the exterior of the gloves on their removal. Gloves should never be reused in first world health care settings where gloves are always readily available.

Cost

In England, health care related infections have been estimated to cost £1,000 million annually (WHO 2005). In June 2009, the DOH estimated some £120 million had been spent on initiatives to attempt to reduce health care related infections. These initiatives together with actions taken by individual NHS Trusts were estimated to have saved between £141 and £263 million in addition to reducing discomfort, distress and deaths that may have been caused by hospital acquired infections (National Audit Office 2009).

Utilizing these approaches in your OSCE examination

An overview of the station

It is likely that you will be asked to demonstrate hand washing or hand decontamination in your OSCE. This may be assessed alone or it may be assessed as a component of another OSCE such as aseptic technique (see Chapter 6). You are advised to check your university guidelines as some may assess this skill formatively using groups of students whilst others may assess individual students using either a summative or formative approach. Whatever the approach the commonalties are:

- You will be asked to demonstrate understanding of effective infection control. This will include:
  - Effective hand washing,
  - Use of alcohol gel to decontaminate hands.
- You will also be questioned on your knowledge related to hand washing and infection control.

The next section provides step by step guidance for each of these areas.

Demonstrating effective hand washing

Step 1

As stated earlier (NPSA 2007) you will need to wet your hands first. This allows a lather to be created and facilitates effective hand washing (see Fig. 5.1a). You should apply sufficient soap to cover all surfaces of the hands.

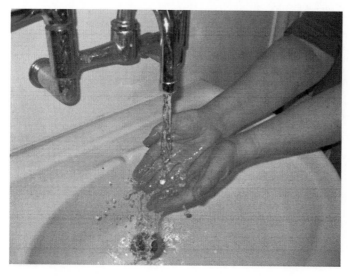

Figure 5.1a Wet your hands before applying soap

Step 2

Once your hands are sufficiently wet you should use the following techniques to clean every area of your hand.

 A video of this technique is included on the online resource centre
www.oxfordtextbooks.co.uk/orc/caballero.

All steps of this process are vital and it is important that you fully understand and are able to demonstrate each step in your OSCE.

- The palms of each hand should be rubbed together as in Fig 5.1b,
- You should then rub the back of each hand with the palm of the other hand with fingers interlaced as in Fig 5.1c,
- You then rub each palm together with fingers interlaced,
- You should then rub the back of your fingers with opposing palms as in Fig 5.1d,
- To clean your thumbs you should rub each thumb clasped in opposite hand using rotational movement as in Fig 5.1e,
- You should then clean your fingertips by rubbing the tips of your fingers in opposite palm in a circular motion as in Fig 5.1f.
- You should finally cleanse your wrist by rubbing each wrist with the opposite hand as in Fig 5.1g.

Step 3

Once you have washed your hands using this technique for approximately 40–60 seconds your hands should then be adequately rinsed under running water, taking care not to contaminate your hands on the tap or the sink as in Fig 5.1h.

Step 4

To prevent recontamination from the taps you should always use your elbows to turn off taps as in Fig 5.1i. Some universities may have taps with sensors; if this is the case there is no need to turn off the taps as they will automatically shut off once you have finished washing your hands. Hands should be dried with a paper towel as in Fig 5.1j.

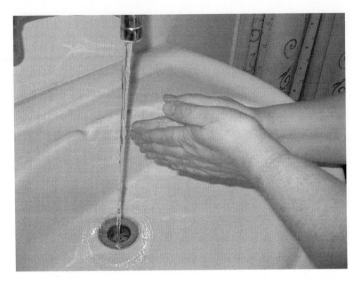

Figure 5.1b Each hand should be rubbed together

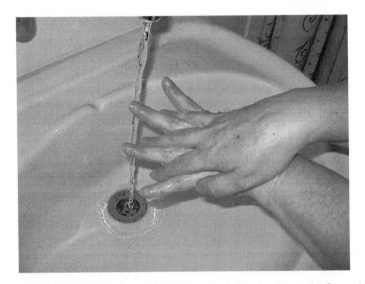

Figure 5.1c Rub the back of each hand with the palm of the other hand with fingers interlaced

Step 5

Hands should now be dried thoroughly with a single use towel and the towel discarded in an appropriate bin. Again you should take care not to contaminate your hands when drying them (see Fig 5.1j).

Hand gel

If you are required to demonstrate using hand gel this should be rubbed in as per manufacturer's guidance.

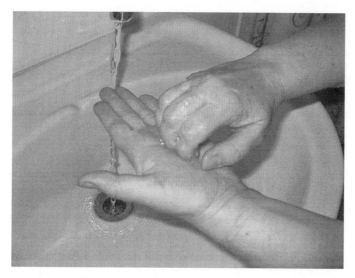

Figure 5.1d Rub the back of your fingers with opposing palms

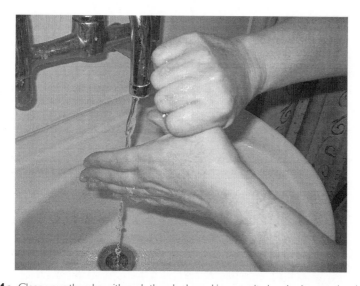

Figure 5.1e Clean your thumbs with each thumb clasped in opposite hand using rotational movement

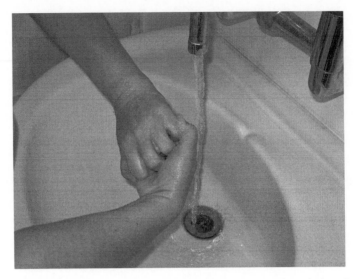

Figure 5.1f Clean fingertips by rubbing the tips of your fingers in opposite palm in a circular motion

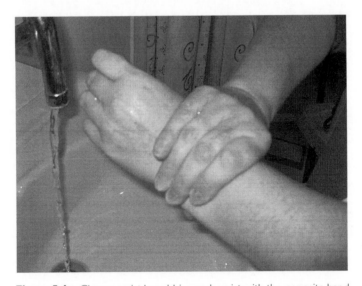

Figure 5.1g Cleanse wrist by rubbing each wrist with the opposite hand

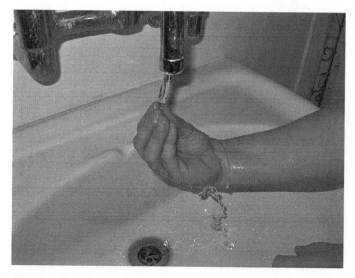

Figure 5.1h Take care not to contaminate hands on the tap or the sink

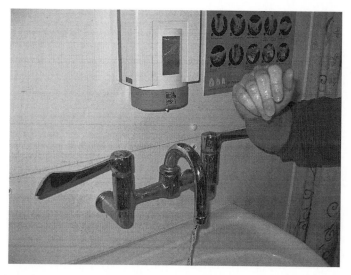

Figure 5.1i Prevent recontamination from the taps by always using your elbows to turn off taps

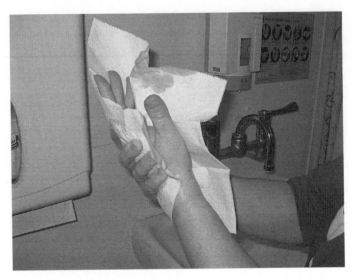

Figure 5.1j Hand drying

 Examiners' marking criteria

Table 5.1 shows typical marking typical marking criteria for this OSCE.

Table 5.1 **Example of examiners' marking criteria**

Student's name and cohort year	
Expected performance criteria	Demonstrated Yes/No
Student is not wearing false nails or nail polish. Nails are short and clean.	
Student is following the bare below the elbows guidance and is not wearing a wrist watch or any item of jewellry or clothing below the level of the elbow.	
Taps are turned on to allow adequate water to flow over hands but not so fast that splashing occurs.	
Water temperature is checked to ensure prolonged rinsing is possible.	
All surfaces of the hands are wet.	
Sufficient soap to cover all surfaces of the hands is applied.	
• Hands are rubbed palm to palm, • Rubs back of each hand with palm of other hand with fingers interlaced, • Hands are rubbed palm to palm with fingers interlaced, • Hands are rubbed with backs of fingers to opposing palms with fingers interlaced,	

Table 5.1 (*continued*)

Student's name and cohort year	
Expected performance criteria	Demonstrated Yes/No
<ul><li>Each thumb is clasped in opposite hand and rotated,</li><li>Tips of fingers are rubbed in palm of opposite hand in circular motion,</li><li>Each wrist is rubbed with opposite hand,</li><li>Both hands are rinsed from fingers to wrist,</li><li>Hands are dried thoroughly using paper towels from fingers to wrists.</li></ul>	
Taps are turned off using elbows.	
Hands are dried thoroughly using paper towels from fingers to wrists.	
Paper towels are dropped into opened bin without contaminating hands.	

Some universities may assess your knowledge in relation to infection control and hand hygiene and it is useful to prepare for that if that is a requirement. Some typical questions are included here. Answers are found in the appendix of this chapter.

Examiners' questions

Typical questions that the examiner might ask are provided in Box 5.1.

Box 5.1 Typical examiners' questions

1. What is meant by the term HAI?
2. What is meant by the term 'microbe'?
3. When should hand hygiene be performed?
4. When should hands be cleaned using soap and water?
5. When may hands be cleaned using alcohol rub?
6. How long should a hand wash take using soap and water?
7. How long should a hand wash take using alcohol rub?
8. When should an antiseptic soap be used?
9. What advantage do antiseptic hand wash solutions have over non-antiseptic soap?
10. Why are bars of soap not advocated for the health care setting?
11. If bars of soap are the only cleaning material available, what precautions should be taken?
12. How many deaths per annum are currently attributed to HAIs in the UK?
13. When should non-sterile gloves be worn?
14. When should sterile gloves be worn?

15. Why should hands be cleaned prior to putting on gloves?
16. Why should hands be cleaned after the removal of gloves?
17. What is the current advocated cost of HAIs in the UK?

Answers are provided at the end of the chapter.

✗ Common errors at this station

- Students do not follow the bare below the elbows guidance,
- Students frequently apply soap before wetting hands,
- Students run tap water too slowly to thoroughly rinse hands,
- Students run water too fast and cause splashing,
- Students fail to wash hands for the advocated time,
- Students fail to complete each of the advocated manoeuvres,
- Students turn off taps with their bare hands,
- Students dry hands rubbing towel from above wrists back to hand.

Online resource centre

You can find further advice and revision help for your OSCEs including a video for this skill by going online now to see **www.oxfordtextbooks.co.uk/orc/caballero/**.

≋ References

Bandolier, (2006). Risk of death from hospital acquired infection in the UK. http://www.medicine.ox.ac.uk/bandolier/booth/Risk/HAI.html accessed 4th February 2011.

Burd, M. (2006). Hygiene in hand. *World of Irish Nursing & Midwifery*, June: 31–32.

Department of Health (2007). Uniforms and workwear: an evidence base for developing local policy. London: Department of Health. http://www.dh.gov.uk/publications accessed 4th February 2011.

Gould, D. (2009). Infection control: hand hygiene. *British Journal of Healthcare Assistants*, 3, 3: 110–113.

www.hpa.org.uk accessed 4th February 2011. www.dh/gov.uk/pandemicflu accessed 4th February 2011.

Health Protection Agency (2011). http://www.hpa.org.uk/Topics/InfectiousDiseases/InfectionsAZ/Handwashing/ accessed 4th February 2011.

Horton, R. (1999). Handwashing: the fundamental infection control principle. *British Journal of Nursing*, 4, 16: 929–933.

National Audit Office (2009). Reducing Healthcare Associated Infections in Hospitals in England, Executive Summary. www.nao.org.uk accessed 4th February 2011.

National Patient Safety Agency (2007). Clean your hands campaign. www.npsa.nhs.uk/cleanyourhands accessed 4th February 2011.

Nazarko, L. (2008). Standard precautions: how to help prevent infection. *British Journal of Healthcare Assistants*, March, 02, 03: 119–123.

Nice (2003). *Infection Control and Prevention of Healthcare-Associated Infections in Primary and Community Care*. London: NICE

Parker, L. (1999). Importance of hand washing in the prevention of cross infection. *British Journal of Nursing*, 8, 11: 716–720.

World Health Organization (2005). *Guidelines on Hand Hygiene in Health Care (Advanced Draft): A Summary*. Geneva: World Health Organization.

World Health Organization (2006). *My 5 Moments for Hand Hygiene*. Geneva: World Health Organization.
World Health Organization (2009). *Guideline on Hand Hygiene in Health Care*. Geneva: World Health Organization.

Appendix: answers to examiners' questions

1. The DOH defines the term HAI as 'healthcare associated infection; this term covers 'any infection by any infectious agent acquired as a consequence of a person's treatment by the NHS or which is acquired by a health care worker in the course of their NHS duties.'

2. A microbe is a living organism that may only be seen with a microscope and cannot be seen with the naked eye.

3. Hand hygiene should be performed in line with the WHO 'My 5 Moments of Hand Hygiene'.

4. Soap and water should be used when hands are visibly soiled, where there has been contact with body fluid or where exposure to spore forming bacteria is suspected.

5. When hands are visibly clean.

6. The WHO recommends 40–60 seconds.

7. The WHO recommends 20–30 seconds.

8. In high risk situations, e.g. prior to invasive procedures, prior to use of aseptic technique, when in contact with patients with reduced defence to infection.

9. Antiseptic solutions are bactericidal and some continue to kill bacteria after hand washing.

10. Soap may harbour microorganisms.

11. If bars of soap are used they should be used for one patient only and allowed to dry between use.

12. Approximately 5,000 deaths per year are attributed to HACIs in the UK (WHO 2005).

13. Non-sterile gloves should be worn when handling any body fluid or where there is a risk of contact with body fluid.

14. Sterile gloves should be worn when there is a break or potential break in the body's integument or when bypassing the body's natural defences, e.g. when passing a urinary catheter.

15. Health care workers have been found to colonize bacteria for prolonged periods of time (WHO 2009) and so care should be taken to ensure minimum contamination.

16. There is always a risk of gloves being punctured, hands may be contaminated on removal, hands sweat and bacteria may move from under nails while hands are contained within gloves.

17. Current cost of HAIs to the NHS in the UK is estimated to be £1,000 million per annum.

Chapter 6
Aseptic non-touch technique (ANTT)

Catherine Caballero

Chapter aims

This chapter will enable you to:

- Revise key material in relation to this skill,
- Follow a step by step guide to the aseptic technique,
- Understand how to prepare and revise for this OSCE,
- Highlight common problems at this station and identify how these may be avoided.

Introduction

During the aseptic technique simulated examination students may be asked to demonstrate a clinical skill, usually a wound dressing, using an aseptic technique. This is becoming increasingly common in all universities as it has been identified as a mandatory simulated assessment in the essential skills clusters (NMC 2007).

This skill is probably one of the most complex skills assessed during simulation and it is vital that students understand the principles of aseptic non-touch technique and are able to demonstrate application of these principles throughout the examination.

Revision of this key material will enable the student to understand and apply the key principles of aseptic non-touch technique throughout the examination.

Key revision for your simulated examination

Nosocomial

This is defined as an infection acquired in hospital at least 72 hours after admission to hospital caused or precipitated whilst the patient is in hospital. Health care acquired infections (HAIs) have become a serious concern over recent years, costing the NHS an estimated £1 billion a year and contributing to some 5,000 deaths a year (Aziz 2009). One factor that has been identified as impacting on the increase in HAIs is the variation of techniques used in wound care. Two of the most common HAIs of recent times are MRSA (methicillin resistant *Staphylococcus aureus*) and C. Diff (*Clostridium difficile*). MRSA is a species of bacterium commonly found on the skin and/or in the noses of healthy people. Although it is usually harmless at these sites, it may occasionally get into the body (e.g. through breaks in the skin such as abrasions, cuts, wounds, surgical incisions or indwelling catheters) and cause infections. These infections may be mild (e.g. pimples or boils) or serious (e.g. infection of the bloodstream, bones or joints). C. Diff is a species of bacterium that causes diarrhoea and other intestinal disease when competing bacterium are wiped out by antibiotics. This bacterium can have major consequences for patients once contracted. However, a number of less profiled infections are contributing to the rise in HAIs e.g. urinary tract infection.

Aspetic non-touch technique (ANTT) is the term given to carrying out procedures which require attention to minimizing the risk of cross contamination that could potentially lead to an infection. Rowley (2001) first identified the ANTT as a way of standardizing the process of aseptic technique used in clinical practice. Aziz (2009: 29) states that the aims of the ANTT are to:

- Improve aseptic technique in the NHS,
- Standardize aseptic technique in the NHS,
- Protect patients by reducing HAIs.

Definition

The term **asepsis** means the absence of any infectious agents such as pathogenic microorganisms (disease producing). However, as we do not live or work in environments where this is routinely possible we use the **aseptic technique** as a means of achieving asepsis, as close as we can. Aseptic techniques prevent cross contamination of wounds and other susceptible sites by organisms that could cause infection. In the literature you will find many ways in which the ANTT is carried out to reduce the risk of cross contamination during clinical procedures but there are three main principles to which you must always adhere. These are:

Never contaminate:

- Yourself,
- Your equipment,
- Your patient.

This can be achieved by ensuring all key parts of the procedure are free from contaminates. Key parts are usually parts of equipment which come into direct contact with the patient's internal structures (Rowley 2001), e.g. sterile gloved hand, dressings, swabs and irrigation equipment in simple wound cleansing and/or dressing. If these key parts are contaminated by infectious materials there is an increase in the risk of infection.

When should an ANTT be used?

The ANTT must be used during any invasive procedure that bypasses the body's natural defence mechanisms, e.g. the skin or mucous membranes (Dougherty and Lister 2008). These procedures include:

- Catheterization,
- Wound cleansing/dressing changes of clean or dirty wounds,
- Removal of sutures/clips/drains etc.,
- Intravenous dressings (IV),
- Total Parenteral Nutrition (TPN),
- Intravenous (IV) drug administration.

There is some debate in the nursing literature as to the effectiveness of using an ANTT for all procedures; however, if there is a potential risk that the patient may acquire an infection during the procedure an ANTT *must* be used. It is important that each patient is assessed for the probability of acquiring an infection—in effect an infection risk assessment. You may then want to think about the patient's immune status, nutritional status, age and/or medical condition (Xavier 1999).

Principles of the ANTT

The six main principles of the ANTT are:

1. Being aware of sources of contamination,
2. Keeping the environment free from pathogens,
3. Effective hand decontamination,
4. Creating a sterile field,
5. Exclusive use of sterilized equipment,
6. Using a non-touch technique.

Being aware of sources of contamination It is vitally important that you are aware of sources of contamination in the clinical setting. These can be from:

- Not washing your hands,
- Not cleaning your trolley or surfaces properly,
- Out of date or contaminated sterile equipment,
- Touching sterile equipment with non-sterile equipment or hands,
- Touching your sterile field with contaminated materials.

Or airborne contamination such as:

- Dust from bed making/cleaning,
- Droplets,
- Nebulizers/humidifiers,
- Air conditioning,
- Sneezing and coughing,
- Open windows and fans.

Keeping the environment free from pathogens It is essential when carrying out the ANTT for wound cleansing and dressing that you pay particular attention to the environment as bacteria are dispersed into the air by a number of practices. For example, close windows, turn off fans and carry out the wound cleaning and dressing once the dust has settled following cleaning and bed making.

Effective hand decontamination Is essential to reduce the risk of cross contamination. The recognized Royal College of Nursing (RCN) (2004) and the National Patient Safety Agency (NPSA) (2008) hand washing technique should be used at the beginning and end of every ANTT (see Chapter 5 and Fig 6.1a).

Creating a sterile field This includes preparing your area and using the appropriate materials. In an **acute** setting a dressing trolley should be made available for you to do this as this enables transfer of materials with ease, thus reducing the risk of contamination. However, they are not essential as any impermeable clean surface can be used as a platform for your sterile field to be laid. Initially clean the dressing trolley with soap and water (see Fig. 6.1b) as this will not only clean any visible dirt/dust

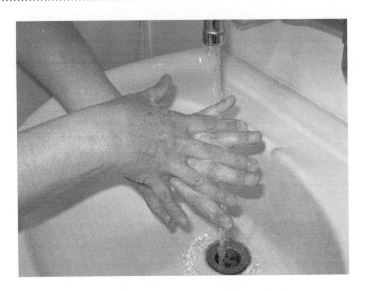

Figure 6.1a Hand washing

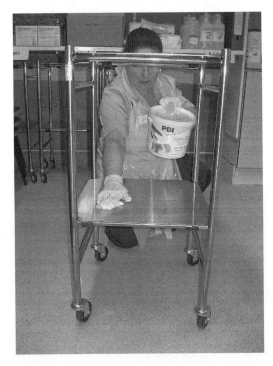

Figure 6.1b Cleaning a trolley with soap solution

but also remove the C. Diff spores which are not killed by 70% alcohol. Following this, clean the trol-ley with a 70% alcohol solution to kill any remaining microorganisms (Pratt *et al.* 2007) (see Fig 6.1c).

Then once you have opened your sterile dressing pack, using fingertips only around the edge, you have a sterile field on which to work (see Fig. 6.1d). If, however, you are in a community setting this is more difficult to achieve (Hallett 2000) and it is necessary for you to either clean an item of the patient's furniture (with their consent) or devise a surface suitable to place your sterile material on and so minimize the possibility of contamination from microorganisms.

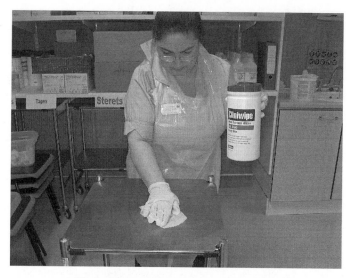

Figure 6.1c Cleaning a trolley with alcohol

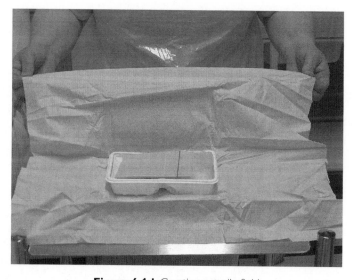

Figure 6.1d Creating a sterile field

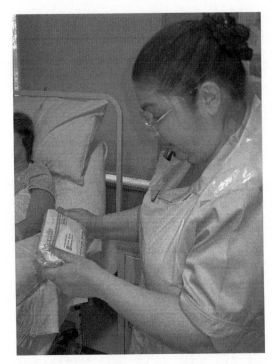

Figure 6.1e Checking sterile equipment

Exclusive use of sterilized equipment   As the main goal of the ANTT is to minimize the risk of cross contamination it is essential that all equipment to be used for the wound cleansing and/or dressing is sterile. Each piece of equipment will come in packaging, which ensures the internal equipment is sterile. It is your responsibility when using this equipment to check for its expiry date and ensure the outer packaging has not been tampered with or damaged, thus potentially making the internal equipment contaminated (see Fig. 6.1e). If you come across outdated or potentially contaminated equipment discard it immediately or inform the manufacturers if a manufacturing problem.

Using a non-touch technique   This is used to prevent direct and indirect contact of key parts of equipment which if touched either directly or indirectly could result in infection (Rowley 2001).

It is therefore essential to carry out a risk assessment prior to carrying out a procedure to ensure you choose the appropriate equipment to minimize the risk of contamination (Preston 2005).

Personal protective clothing

❗ *Note:* It is necessary for you when carrying out the ANTT in wound dressing that you wear ❗
the appropriate protective clothing.

In relation to simple wound cleansing and dressing you only need to wear a single use disposable apron, a pair of non-sterile gloves to remove the old dressing, and sterile gloves to carry out the wound cleansing and dressing (see Fig. 6.1f). If, however, there is a risk of splashing of bodily fluids you may be required to wear other protective clothing such as masks and goggles (Hart 2007). As you progress through your pre-registration programme the wound cleansing and dressings will become more complex and the risk of splashing of bodily fluids may increase.

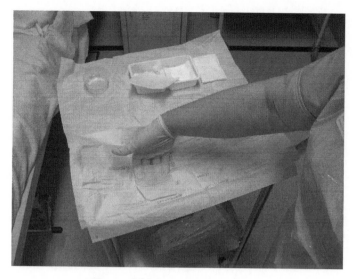

Figure 6.1f Putting on sterile gloves

Box 6.1 **Remember**

1. Effective hand decontamination is the single most effective way of preventing cross contamination.
2. 'The first priority of any non-emergency clinical procedure is to ensure safe aseptic practice' (Rowley and Simon 2009: 23).
3. Always use the ANTT when there is a risk of cross contamination and you will **never** contaminate yourself, equipment or patient.

Wound assessment

One of the things you will be expected to do during your OSCE is to assess the wound. The examiner will expect you to assess the need for the wound to be cleansed and for you to be able to recognize signs of infection (see Fig. 6.1g).

✱ KEY POINT! Not all wounds need to be cleansed and there is evidence (Tomlinson 1987) that cleaning wounds ritualistically can be damaging to new tissue growth. Therefore wound cleansing should only be carried out if the wound is visibly dirty or there are signs of infection, i.e. local redness, swelling or pain etc.

If signs of infection are present a wound swab will need to be taken before cleansing begins. You will also need to identify if the wound has a **localized infection,** i.e. one that is contained in one area, or a **systemic infection,** i.e. one that has spread throughout the body. The type of wound will also enable you to decipher if you are going to irrigate the wound or use swabs to clean the edges of a wound.

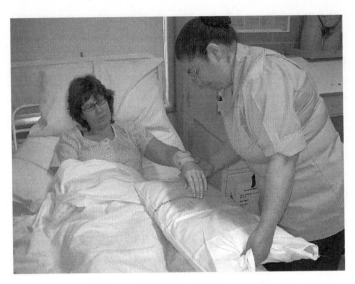

Figure 6.1g Assessing the wound

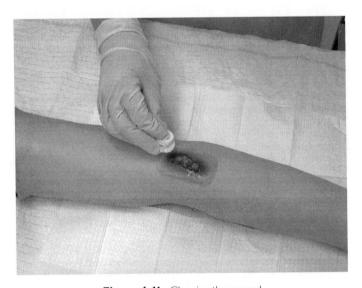

Figure 6.1h Cleaning the wound

Wound cleansing

You will be expected to clean the wound during your OSCE to demonstrate your ability to clean a wound whilst maintaining an aseptic non-touch technique (see Fig. 6.1h).

The aim of wound cleansing is to remove foreign material, e.g. dead tissue, microorganisms causing infection, faecal or urine contamination.

Irrigation of the wound should be used when there is exposed tissue, e.g. pressure sore, leg ulcer or lacerations. Swabs may be used for the removal of physical matter but be mindful that using gauze swabs may serve to redistribute bacteria and could also damage granulating skin and therefore delay

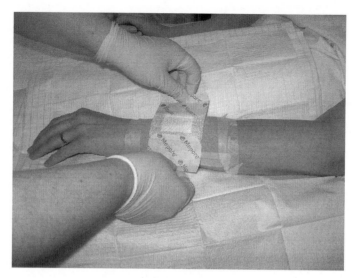

Figure 6.1i Dressing the wound

healing (Tomlinson 1987). In addition, small particles of gauze/cotton wool balls may be left in the wound, thus creating an area for bacteria growth. Swabs, however, can be used to clean the edges of closed wounds, e.g. surgical wounds.

✳ KEY POINT! Wounds should be exposed for the shortest time possible to prevent contamination from airborne materials.

It is recommended by Xavier (1999) that when you are faced with a patient who has more than one wound, the clean non-infected wound should be cleaned first to prevent cross contamination of infected material passing to a clean wound. However, if you are using the principles of the ANTT then cross contamination should not happen whichever wound you clean first. Once the wound is clean and dry apply an appropriate sterile dressing (see Fig. 6.1i).

Dressing a wound is a very complex skill that is difficult to depict in its entirety by still photographs.

 To increase your understanding a video of the procedure and a PowerPoint presentation are available on the online resource centre:
www.oxfordtextbooks.co.uk/orc/caballero/

The video includes step by step guides and includes:

- Introduction to asepsis,
- Setting up of the procedure,
- Carrying out the procedure,
- Post procedural responsibilities.

The OSCE is likely to be performed in a clinical skills laboratory at your university campus, and you will generally have a time limit of between 20 and 30 minutes to complete the skill. The room will be set up with a bed and a patient who could be either a manikin, a volunteer from outside the university, or a member of the wider teaching staff from your university school of nursing. In addition the room will have all the relevant equipment for you to carry out the procedure, such as dressing packs, aprons and gloves.

You will be expected to talk to the 'patient', gain their consent and ask any other relevant questions. You will then be expected to carry out a simple wound cleansing procedure, wound assessment and dressing change. Following the completion of the procedure you may be asked some questions about the ANTT or infection control issues so be prepared!

 # Examiners' marking criteria

The criteria used to assess your aseptic non-touch technique will vary between universities and will depend upon the type of wound that you are dressing. An example of simulated examination criteria is given in Table 6.1.

Table 6.1 **Example of examiners' marking criteria**

Student's name and cohort year	
Expected performance criteria	Demonstrated Yes/No
Student complies with infection control dress code policy—hair off collar, short sleeves, no wrist watches and only one plain wedding band where institutional policy allows.	
Student checks documentation or care plan for recommended procedure and dressing.	
Student negotiates with the patient a suitable time to undertake the dressing, explains procedure to patient and gains consent.	
Student checks if patient requires any analgesia prior to procedure.	
Student leaves patient to prepare equipment.	
Student closes any open windows.	
Student cleans hands.	
Student cleans trolley with soap wipe (where applicable) and 70% spirit or alcohol wipes.	
Student places all equipment on bottom of trolley: Check list: Dressing pack, sterile water/saline, disposable/sterile gloves, scissors/sterile scissors, alcohol wipe, dressing, tape, apron. Cleans outside of saline sachet/ampoule and scissors if required. Removes outer layer of tape.	
Student brings trolley to bed area by holding legs, then screens the bed and ensures patient is in a comfortable position and there is easy access to the dressing site.	
Student ensures easy access to the bed area. Raises or lowers the bed to an appropriate height for them to work.	

Table 6.1 (*continued*)

Student's name and cohort year	
Expected performance criteria	Demonstrated Yes/No
Student checks patient, repeats explanation, cleans hands, puts on apron and loosens dressing tape (non-sterile gloves may be worn).	
Student cleans hands.	
Student places trolley in a convenient position to complete dressing.	
Student checks pack for expiry date and checks it is sterile. Then opens pack and slides contents on to top shelf.	
Student opens sterile field using outer corners only.	
Student places hand in disposable bag and arranges contents of dressing pack.	
Student removes used dressing with bag and then inverts bag and secures to trolley.	
Student checks other packs for expiry dates and sterility and tips onto centre of sterile field.	
Student cleans hands.	
Student puts on sterile gloves, taking care to maintain sterility.	
Student cleans wound if appropriate.	
Student applies clean dressing and secures.	
Student removes gloves.	
Student disposes of waste appropriately in clinical bag, seals bag and places on top of trolley.	
Student cleans hands.	
Student checks patient's comfort. Lowers bed, places buzzer etc. within reach of patient and cleans hands before leaving bed area.	
Student removes screens.	
Student disposes of all equipment appropriately.	
Student cleans trolley.	
Student washes hands with soap and water.	
Student documents all care given.	

Examiners' questions

! *Note:* Some universities may assess your knowledge in relation to aseptic non-touch technique and it is useful to prepare for that, if it is a requirement. !

Some typical questions are included in Box 6.2.

Box 6.2 Example of examiners' questions

1. What is asepsis?
2. What is an aseptic technique?
3. When should an aseptic technique be used?
4. Identify four principles of asepsis.
5. What is a nosocomial infection?
6. What are the consequences of nosocomial infection?
7. What are the most common nosocomial infections?
8. What is a non-touch technique?
9. What signs might indicate that a wound is infected?
10. What is a localized infection?
11. What is a systemic infection?
12. What are the three most common ways of spreading infection?
13. Why should you wear protective clothing?
14. What can cause airborne contamination?
15. What should you clean a dressing trolley with?

See the end of the chapter for answers.

✗ Common errors at this station

A number of errors occur at this station. These include failure to:

- Introduce yourself to the patient,
- Gain consent from the patient,
- Check patient documentation or care plan for recommended procedure and dressing,
- Check windows are shut/check for cross contamination,
- Follow university/NHS Trust dress code,
- Check need for analgesia,
- Clean trolley effectively,
- Dispose of equipment appropriately,
- Prevent contamination of sterile field:
    - Placing non-sterile equipment on sterile field,
    - Touching field with uniform/hands,

- Placing 'dirty' equipment/dressings on sterile field.
- Prevent contamination of sterile equipment:
  - Gloves touched and contaminated,
  - Touching equipment whilst opening packages,
  - Forgetting which bits of equipment are sterile/not sterile.
- Carry out correct wound cleaning techniques,
- Decontaminate hands or more commonly too frequent hand decontamination,
- Carry out appropriate glove technique and contamination of gloves,
- Avoid ripping gloves,
- Avoid panicking if mistake made and trying to cover up.

✚ Top tips for passing this station

- Practise, practise, practise the procedure prior to taking the OSCE, using any resources your university provides such as DVDs, and skills laboratories. In addition practise under the direct supervision of your mentor whilst on clinical placements.

- You could mock up a sterile pack at home by using a tea towel as your sterile field, an egg cup as your fluid receptacle, some kitchen paper as sterile gauze and a pair of household rubber gloves as sterile gloves and follow the DVD step by step to develop your ability to carry out the procedure.

- Revise the underpinning knowledge in relation to this station as you may be asked questions at the end of carrying out the procedure. Please refer to the section on questions in this chapter to guide your revision.

- If during the OSCE you rip or contaminate your gloves or any aspect of your sterile field do not panic; just stop, explain to the examiner what you have done and start again.

- If you need to start again be aware that you may well be under a time constraint but again do not panic carry out the procedure as best you can.

- If you run out of time you will be referred (i.e. not passed yet) at this attempt but be assured it is better you run out of time rather than not recognize a contamination of the sterile field.

- If you are referred (i.e. not passed yet) at your first attempt do not panic; you will be given another opportunity to pass.

- If you pass, congratulations—you have mastered one of the most fundamental techniques that underpin your nursing practice.

@ Online resource centre

You can find further advice and revision help for your OSCEs by going online now to see **www.oxfordtextbooks.co.uk/orc/caballero/**.

≋ References

Aziz, A.M. (2009). Variations in aseptic technique and implications for infection control. *British Journal of Nursing*, 18, 1: 26–31.

Dougherty, L. and Lister, S. (eds) (2008). *The Royal Marsden Hospital Manual of Clinical Nursing Procedures.* 7th edn. Oxford: Blackwell Publishing.

Hallett, C. (2000). Infection control in wound care: a study of fatalism in community nursing. *Journal of Clinical Nursing,* 9: 103–109.

Hart, S. (2007). Using an aseptic technique to reduce the risk of infection. *Nursing Standard,* 21, 47: 43–48.

National Patient Safety Agency (2008). Clean hands save lives. Patient Safety Alert ref 0773 2nd edn. 2nd September, www. npsa.nhs.uk.

NMC (2007). Essential Skills Clusters. London: NMC.

Pratt, R.J., Pellowe, C.M., Wilson, J.A., Loveday, H.P., Harper, P.J., Jones, S.R.L.J., McDougall, C. and Wilcox, M.H., (2007). Epic 2. National evidence based guidelines for preventing health care associated infection in NHS hospitals in England. *Journal of Hospital Infection* 65S: S1–S64.

Preston, R.M. (2005). Aseptic technique: evidence-based approach for patient safety. *British Journal of Nursing,* 14, 10: 540–546.

Rowley, S. (2001). Aseptic non-touch technique. *Nursing Times Plus,* 97, 7: PV1–V111.

Rowley, S. and Simon, C. (2009). Improving standards of aseptic practice through an ANTT trust-wide implementation process: a matter of prioritization and care. *Journal of Infection Prevention,* September, 10, Supplement 1.

Royal College of Nursing (2004). *Hand Washing Technique Poster.* London: RCN. Publication code: 002 277.

Tomlinson, D. (1987). To clean or not to clean? Cleaning discharging surgical wounds. *Nursing Times,* 83, (9): 71, 73, 75.

Xavier, G. (1999). Asepsis. *Nursing Standard,* 13, 36: 49–53.

💬 Appendix: answers to examiners' questions

1. What is asepsis?
   - Freedom from pathogenic microorganisms,
   - The absence of disease producing microorganisms.

2. What is an aseptic technique?
   - A collective term of methods used to maintain asepsis and designed to interrupt the transmission of infection.
   - A technique that reduces the risk of cross contamination during clinical procedures.
   - Effort taken to keep patient as free from microorganisms as possible.
   - Method to prevent cross contamination of wounds and other susceptible sites by organisms that could cause infection.
   - The prevention of microbial contamination of living tissue or fluid or sterile materials by excluding, removing or killing microorganisms.

3. When should an aseptic technique be used?
   Any invasive procedure that bypasses the body's natural defences, e.g.
   - Catheterization,
   - Dressings,
   - Removal of sutures/clips etc.
   - IV dressings,
   - TPN,
   - IV drug administration.

4. Identify four principles of asepsis.
   - Effective hand decontamination,
   - Creating a sterile field,
   - Exclusive use of sterilized equipment,
   - Using a non-touch technique,
   - Being aware of sources of contamination,
   - Keeping environment free from pathogens.

5. What is a nosocomial infection?
  * A hospital acquired infection,
  * An infection not present on admission.

6. What are the consequences of nosocomial infection?
  * Financial cost to the NHS Trust,
  * Increased patient days in hospital,
  * Increased morbidity,
  * Increased mortality,
  * Pain,
  * Inconvenience to patient,
  * Increased hospital waiting lists,
  * Increased suffering of patient.

7. What are the most common nosocomial infections?
  * Catheter related infections,
  * Surgical sites,
  * Pneumonias,
  * Bloodstream (IV lines).
  * MRSA
  * *C. Diff*

8. What is a non-touch technique?
  A technique that prevents contamination of the area by microorganisms on the hands. It involves the following:
  * Always wash hands effectively,
  * Never contaminate key parts,
  * Touch non-key parts with confidence,
  * Take appropriate infective precautions,
  * Maintain asepsis and a non-touch approach.

9. What signs might indicate that a wound is infected?
  * Local redness,
  * Swelling,
  * Pain,
  * Pyrexia,
  * Increased white cell count.

10. What is a localized infection?
  * Infection that is contained in one area, e.g. wound.

11. What is a systemic infection?
  * Infection that has spread throughout the body.

12. What are the three most common ways of spreading infection?
  * Poor hand hygiene,
  * Inanimate objects,
  * Dust particles.

13. Why should you wear protective clothing?
  * Protection from splashes during procedure,
  * Protection from direct contact during procedure,
  * Protection of skin and clothing during procedure,
  * Prevent transfer of pathogens from nurse to patient,
  * Prevent nurse acquiring infection from patient.

14. What can cause airborne contamination?
  * Bed making,
  * Cleaning,

- Droplets,
- Nebulizers/humidifiers,
- Air conditioning,
- Sneezing,
- Coughing.

15. What should you clean a dressing trolley with?
    - 70% ethanol alcohol.

Chapter 7
Measuring, assessing and recording: pulse, body temperature, respirations and oxygen saturation

Paula Deamer and Tina Attoe

Chapter aims

This chapter will enable you to:

- Revise key material in relation to physiological assessment,
- Follow a step by step guide to each observation,
- Understand how to prepare and revise for this OSCE,
- Highlight common questions and problems at this station and identify how these may be avoided.

Introduction

As part of the measuring physical observations simulated examination, students will be asked to measure, assess and record pulse, body temperature, respirations and oxygen saturation. This assessment is becoming more common in all universities as it has been identified as a mandatory simulated assessment within the NMC Essential Skills Clusters (NMC 2007).

Although this chapter will focus upon each observation in turn, it is imperative that when undertaking physical observations the findings are not assessed in isolation. Like a jigsaw, each result, alongside the patient's appearance, pallor, demeanour and responsiveness, link together to form an overall picture of the patient's condition. The skill of undertaking these observations may sometimes be reviewed as being routine, but the skill has important clinical significance. Students have to demonstrate their underpinning knowledge and to make sense of the relevance of the observations—this can be complex and challenging. Some student nurses will have previous experience, prior to commencing their nurse education training, of taking patients' physical observations, but the ability to demonstrate an understanding of the underpinning knowledge differentiates between the role of a health care support worker and a student nurse.

Revision of key material will enable the student to understand, undertake and assess the relevance of measuring pulse, body temperature, respirations and oxygen saturation. The importance of the professional nurse's ability to accurately assess, record and evaluate pulse rate, body temperature, respirations and oxygen saturation cannot be underestimated.

Concern has been raised that NHS staff are failing to recognize patient deterioration in a timely manner. In a study by the National Patient Safety Agency (NPSA 2007) factors for this lack of recognition included failure to take physical observations, not acknowledging the significance of the observations and finally not reporting on issues that were of concern, or acting upon these findings. Guidelines on recognizing and managing patient deterioration have been issued by NICE (2007) along-side competencies for recognition and management of a deteriorating patient, which all staff working in acute settings should achieve (DOH 2009). Throughout these the importance of assessing, record-ing, evaluating and appropriately reacting to the results of physical observations cannot be denied.

When undertaking all observations a student nurse should have an awareness of the standard acceptable ranges of the physical assessment measurements. The first recorded measurements are frequently referred to as the patient's baseline readings. Each individual will have their own unique baseline measurements, which are normal for them. Physical measurements are influenced by life-style, age, personal fitness levels, diet, alcohol consumption and cigarette smoking. The baseline measurement results allow the nurse to make a more accurate judgement about the observation findings based upon specific individual circumstances.

> *Note:* If a patient is stressed due to hospital admission, being in pain or from the influence of a disease process this may also cause the baseline measurements to be outside the acceptable ranges. Therefore, the student should have knowledge of the acceptable range for each of the observations in order to aid evaluation and recognition of abnormal findings.

Key revision for your simulated examination

Measuring, assessing and recording pulse rate

Pulse rate is considered to be one of the four vital signs of life alongside blood pressure, body tempera-ture and respiratory rate. A pulse is created by a pressure wave being generated throughout the arte-rial system, following the expansion and recoil of the arteries with each contraction of the left ventricle (Marieb and Hoehn 2007). Fingertip compression of the artery against the underlying bone will enable the pulse to be located; this action is called palpation. The pulse indicates that the heart is pumping and moving blood around the body to perfuse the tissues (Diggens 2009). Therefore, absence of a pulse may indicate that the heart is not pumping or blood is not reaching the peripheries.

There are a number of sites which can be utilized to measure pulse; however, when completing physical observations the **radial pulse is** commonly used, since it is easily accessed and the pulse at this site, in healthy individuals, has a discernable strength. Table 7.1 outlines the indications for using specific pulse sites.

Guidance for effective measurement of the pulse

> *Note:* Remember to wash your hands prior to undertaking this skill. If there is a risk that your patient may have an infection you should consider wearing gloves and apron, in accordance with local policy guidelines.

The pulse is measured by palpation of the radial artery by placing the index and middle fingertip pads along the radial artery in line with the base of the patient's thumb whilst simultaneously counting the number of beats felt during one timed minute (see Fig. 7.1). Sufficient pressure to feel the pulse should be applied without causing discomfort. When palpating the pulse you must not place your thumb on the underside of the patient's wrist. The thumb pad has a discernable pulse of its own and

Table 7.1 **Indications for palpating specific pulse sites**

Pulse site	When to use this site
Carotid Central pulse site close to heart—strong pulsation due to being large artery.	Commonly used in sudden deterioration, peripheral shutdown and **cardiac arrest** situations.
Brachial Peripheral pulse site—less palpable strength.	Commonly used when assessing blood pressure, and confirming circulation to the lower arm following surgery or trauma.
Radial Peripheral pulse site—less palpable strength and easily accessible.	Most commonly used pulse site in clinical practice for assessing patient's pulse rate.
Femoral Central pulse, close to heart—strong pulsation due to being large artery. Not easily accessed.	Commonly used to assess blood supply to lower limbs, particularly in peripheral vascular disease. If head or neck trauma has occurred this is an alternative site to the carotid pulse.
Popliteal, posterior tibial and dorsalis pedis Peripheral pulse sites much less palpable strength and can be difficult to locate.	Commonly used to assess circulation, particularly in peripheral vascular disease and diabetic peripheral neuropathy and crush injury trauma.

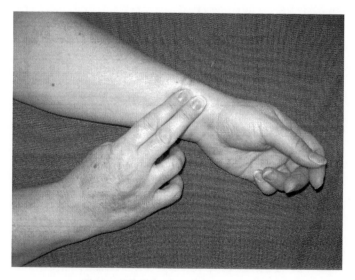

Figure 7.1 Palpation of the radial artery

could be misinterpreted as being the patient's pulse rate. Whilst completing this task you should also assess the rhythm and amplitude of the pulse. This would not be identifiable if using an electronic means to assess the patient's pulse rate. A full minute is required since it allows you to discern subtle changes in rate, rhythm and amplitude (strength) which may be missed if the assessment was completed in a shorter time period.

> Box 7.1 **Ranges for pulse**
>
> 60–100 beats per minute (bpm) normal range,
> < 60 bpm bradycardia (slow pulse),
> > 100 bpm tachycardia (fast pulse).

Pulse rate is expressed as beats per minute. When assessing and evaluating the patient's pulse rate you should have an awareness of the normal acceptable range and the patient's baseline measurement, when obtainable. Box 7.1 identifies normal and abnormal ranges.

Documentation of pulse

It is important to document your findings immediately after taking the patient's pulse, to ensure accuracy. Most clinical care settings will require the documentation to be completed using black ink. Your written documentation will be accessed by all members of the care team and may be utilized to inform patient treatment decisions; therefore it is imperative that your measurements cannot be misinterpreted.

Table 7.2 provides an example of how you would document a patient's pulse which was found to be 124 bpm at 08.00 am. You should document the actual reading in figures as well as placing a clear dot between 120 and 130 where 124 would be approximately located.

! *Note:* Not all care settings will have documentation that differentiates the pulse readings by units of ten. Therefore prior to completing the OSCE you should familiarize yourself with the local documentation. !

Table 7.2 **How to document a patient's pulse**

Pulse (bpm)	01/09/20XX 08.00	Date/ Time	Date/ Time
140			
130			
120	124 .		
110			
100			
90			
80			
70			
60			
50			
40			

In this example the patient's pulse rate is above the acceptable range (indicated in white as between 60 and 100 bpm) and the patient's pulse rate falls within the light grey coloured section; this indicates that the patient's condition could be of concern for the nurse. Note: Some NHS Trusts will not use colour coded charts and you will be expected to score the pulse according to local policy. Whenever a reading is found to be outside the acceptable range you would always be expected to bring this to your mentor's attention and follow local policy regarding actions that should be taken. In this case the patient should be kept under close observation and the pulse rate should be monitored more frequently.

Frequently asked question related to measuring pulse rate

Q) I am unable to locate the radial pulse site.

It is very common when completing this skill that students place their fingers on the inner aspect of the wrist rather than the radial pulse site which is located on the outer aspect. You may also be placing your index and middle fingertip pads too far up the arm.

Many students believe that this is a simple skill and it appears evident that they have not been practising this in the clinical setting, but relying upon electronic means for assessing a patient's pulse rate. You should therefore familiarize yourself with the correct technique and practise this skill before the OSCE, following the guidelines for measuring pulse rate as described in this chapter.

Measuring, assessing and recording body temperature

Body temperature is the balance between heat production and heat loss in response to metabolic reaction within the body. It is possible to measure a patient's surface and core body temperature. For the purpose of this OSCE the reading you obtain will be identified as the core body temperature. The core temperature reading indicates the heat of arterial blood and body tissue heat from metabolic activity. A core body temperature provides the most accurate reading. Surface temperature will be cooler than core body temperature as heat loss occurs through the skin.

> *Note:* The patient's body temperature can be influenced by internal and external factors; therefore significant variances could be an indication that your patient's condition is deteriorating and should be investigated. Like all physical observations, there is an acceptable range for body temperature, and if the patient's temperature was within this range it would not necessarily be a cause of concern. Measurements between 36°C–37.5°C (Centigrade) are all considered to be within the acceptable range (see Box 7.2).

Whilst completing this skill you should be maintaining communication with the patient, and this may assist you to gain more insight into the patient's personal awareness of whether their temperature is normally low or high in relation to the acceptable range. For some patients a measurement that indicates a body temperature of 37.5°C may be acceptable, whereas another patient may state that their usual body temperature is on the lower end of the spectrum and for this patient it may indicate that they are pyrexial. The term **pyrexia** is applied to a patient whose temperature is above the acceptable parameters. There are a number of sites that can be used to measure body temperature, including the ear, the mouth, under the arm and rectally (see Table 7.3). Box 7.2 identifies normal and abnormal ranges.

Guidance for effective measurement of body temperature

To assess a patient's body temperature you can use any one of the many available thermometers, including tympanic, digital or chemical/heat reactive strips, to obtain your reading. Your choice should be influenced by patient condition and the range of available equipment.

Box 7.2 **Ranges for temperature**

Measurements between 36°C and 37.5°C normal range
  < 35.5°C hypothermia (low),
  > 38°C pyrexia (high).

Table 7.3 **Indications for selection of specific temperature sites**

Tympanic Utilizes the tympanic membrane located via the inner ear canal.	A commonly used site, which has easy access and an immediate reading, using a tympanic thermometer.
Oral Utilizes the buccal pouch under the tongue.	A commonly used site using digital and chemical/heat reactive strips.
Axilla Located in the armpit.	Infrequently used due to inaccuracy. The reading takes 3–5 minutes, depending on individual manufacturer's instructions.
Rectal Temperature is measured by inserting the thermometer into the patient's rectum.	Not generally advocated due to invasive nature.

Remember to wash your hands and clean your equipment prior to commencing this skill. If there is a risk that your patient may have an infection or risk of personal contamination you should consider wearing gloves and apron, in accordance with local policy guidelines.

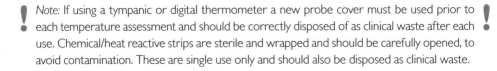 *Note:* If using a tympanic or digital thermometer a new probe cover must be used prior to each temperature assessment and should be correctly disposed of as clinical waste after each use. Chemical/heat reactive strips are sterile and wrapped and should be carefully opened, to avoid contamination. These are single use only and should also be disposed as clinical waste.

Tympanic

Tympanic membrane thermometers are inserted into a patient's ear canal (see Fig. 7.2). The probe must be covered and placed snugly into the patient's ear. The thermometer needs to be close to the tympanic membrane in order to ensure the reading obtained is accurate. Once in position the scan button should be pressed and when an audible beep is omitted this indicates that the temperature has been read.

Oral

Digital   The covered probe is inserted sublingually into the buccal pouch, under the patient's tongue (see Fig. 7.3). The patient should be asked to close their mouth to create a seal. The timing for accurately obtaining a digital temperature may vary according to type of digital thermometer used in the care setting; this can range between a few seconds and a few minutes. You should familiarize yourself with the required timings for your selected digital thermometer before undertaking the skill.

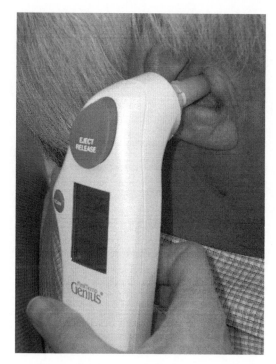

Figure 7.2 Using a tympanic thermometer

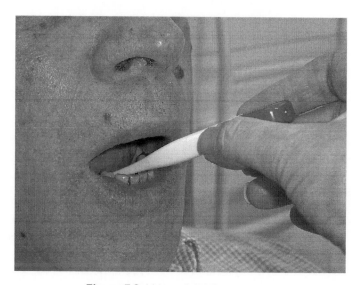

Figure 7.3 Using a digital thermometer

Chemical/heat reactive strips   The chemical/heat reactive strip is also inserted sublingually into the buccal pouch. The patient should be asked to close their mouth and create a seal. The timing for accurately obtaining a temperature using a chemical/heat reactive strip may vary between 1 and 3 minutes (see Fig. 7.4). You should ensure that you are familiar with the manufacturer's instructions prior to commencing this assessment.

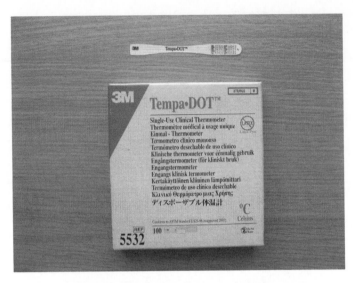

Figure 7.4 Chemical/heat reactive strips

Axilla

Digital   The digital thermometer is inserted into the axilla (armpit). The patient should be asked to place their arm across their chest, to ensure that the digital thermometer is kept in position and therefore enable an accurate reading to be achieved. The timing for accurately obtaining a digital temperature may vary according to type of digital thermometer used in the care setting; this can range between a few seconds and a few minutes. You should familiarize yourself with the required timings for your selected digital thermometer before undertaking the skill.

Chemical/heat reactive strips   The chemical/heat reactive strip can be inserted into the axilla (armpit). The patient should be asked to place their arm across their chest, to ensure that the strip is kept in position and therefore enable an accurate reading to be achieved. The timing for accurately obtaining a temperature using a chemical/heat reactive strip may vary between 1 and 3 minutes. You should ensure that you are familiar with the manufacturer's instructions prior to commencing this assessment.

Documentation of body temperature

> *Note:* It is important to document your findings immediately after measuring the patient's body temperature, to ensure accuracy. Most clinical care settings will require the documentation to be completed using black ink. Your written documentation will be accessed by all members of the care team and may be utilized to inform patient treatment decisions; therefore it is imperative that your measurements cannot be misinterpreted.

Table 7.4 provides an example of how you would document a patient's body temperature that was identified as 37.5°C at 08.00 am. You should document the actual reading in figures as well as placing a clear dot centrally between 37°C and 38°C. Not all care settings will have documentation that differentiates the temperature readings by units of ten; therefore prior to completing the OSCE you should familiarize yourself with the local documentation.

Table 7.4 **How to document a patient's body temperature**

Temp (°C)	01/09/20XX 08.00	Date/ Time	Date/ Time
40.0			
39.0			
38.0			
37.0	37.5 .		
36.0			
35.0			
34.0			
33.0			

In this example the patient's body temperature is within the acceptable range (indicated in white as between 36°C and 37.9°C). Note: Some NHS Trusts will not use colour coded charts and you will be expected to score the temperature according to local policy. The patient's body temperature should not cause any concern to the nurse. However, if a reading is found to be outside the acceptable range the student nurse would always be expected to bring this to their mentor's attention and follow local guidance regarding actions that should be taken. In this case the patient's body temperature would be monitored as per their individual care pathway requirements.

Frequently asked question related to measuring body temperature

Q) Why have I obtained an unexpectedly low tympanic temperature reading, when my patient does not seem to be hypothermic?

Have you ensured that the mode setting of the tympanic thermometer is correctly set for the type of measurement required? It is easy to accidentally change this setting when holding and pressing the scan button. The setting should always be tympanic oral when measuring core body temperature. If the tympanic thermometer has been accidentally set on surface mode the result indicated will be inaccurately low.

If you are nervous your hands may visibly shake and can be felt by the patient or OSCE assessor taking the patient role. This can result in the thermometer not being inserted correctly to gain an accurate reading and invariably you will find that the thermometer indicates a low reading.

! *Note:* Always ensure that you have inserted the tympanic thermometer far enough into the ear, without causing the patient discomfort, to enable the thermometer to detect the true temperature from the tympanic membrane. If this is not done it will also give an inaccurate reading.

Students frequently identify that they have obtained a low reading, e.g. 35.8°C, but are not able to articulate that this is below the acceptable range and what might have caused this low reading. Some students simply state that this is not within the acceptable range. If this happens in your OSCE you should retake the temperature taking into consideration the previously mentioned points.

If the reading remains low you should consider utilizing the other ear and/or using an alternative means of temperature measurement, such as digital or a chemical/heat reactive strip.

You should familiarize yourself with the correct technique and practise this skill before the OSCE, following the guidelines for measuring body temperature as described in this chapter.

Measuring, assessing and recording respiration

Definition

Ventilation is when a patient inhales air into and exhales air from the lungs, a process that facilitates gaseous exchange. Measuring this in nursing is commonly known as assessing respiration. The respiratory system includes the nasal cavity, pharynx, larynx, trachea, bronchi and lungs (Marieb and Hoehn 2007). The purpose of respiration is to supply the body with oxygen during inhalation and remove carbon dioxide by exhalation. During inhalation the diaphragm and external intercostal muscles are contracted causing the rib cage to rise and therefore increasing the volume of the thorax (Marieb and Hoehn 2007). Exhalation is a passive response caused when the muscles relax and the lungs recoil.

Respiration is assessed by observing the rise and fall of the chest and counting each cycle of inhalation and exhalation as one single respiration. This observation must take a full timed minute. Whilst completing this observation you should also be noting the effort, depth and sound of each breath, as well as the patient's pallor. A patient's normal respirations are almost silent. Increased rate and depth of respiration is described as hyperventilation. Any measurement findings that are outside the acceptable range for respiration, as well as any change in the depth, rate and sound of the ventilation process must be reported to a senior member of nursing staff, for close monitoring. You should also assess for good perfusion of oxygen to the skin, by ensuring that the patient's lips and nose do not have a tinge of blue.

Guidance for effective measurement of respiration

To assess a patient's respiration you will need to be able to view the rise and fall of the patient's chest. This is a difficult skill to complete as patients' breathing rates can be affected if they become aware that you are closely monitoring their respiration. Some patients may reduce their respiratory rate, whilst others may increase the number of breaths per minute or exaggerate their respiratory behaviour. A commonly used technique to overcome this is to take the patient's pulse for one minute, maintain the finger positioning for a further minute, and then discreetly count their respiratory rate. Since the patient will be unaware that you are now monitoring their respiration it is more likely that you will obtain an accurate reading. Box 7.3 identifies normal and abnormal ranges.

Box 7.3 Ranges for respiration

Respiratory rate per minute between 11 and 20 normal range
  < 11 bradypnoea (low),
  > 20 tachypnoea (high).

Documentation of respiratory rate

It is important to document your findings immediately after measuring the patient's respiratory rate, to ensure accuracy. Most clinical care settings will require the documentation to be completed using black ink. Your written documentation will be accessed by all members of the care team and may be utilized to inform patient treatment decisions; therefore it is imperative that your measurements cannot be misinterpreted.

Table 7.5 provides an example of how you would document a patient's respiratory rate that was identified as being 13 respirations per minute at 08.00 am. The reading should be documented in figures. There may be differences between each care setting's chart format. Therefore prior to completing the OSCE you should familiarize yourself with the local documentation.

In this example the patient's respiration rate is within the acceptable range (indicated in white as between 11 and 20 respirations per minute). At this point the patient's respirations would not cause any concern. However, if a reading is found to be outside the acceptable range the student nurse would always be expected to bring this to their mentor's attention and follow local policy regarding actions that should be taken. In this case the patient's respirations would be monitored as per their individual care pathway requirements.

Frequently asked questions related to measuring respiratory rate

Q) I feel self conscious watching the rise and fall of a patient's chest.

It is possible to discreetly assess a patient's respiration without staring directly at the patient's chest. By not staring you will feel less self conscious. The patient will not be made to feel uncomfortable and will be less aware of the assessment being completed. This will also result in the respiratory measurement being more accurate.

As you become more skilled at undertaking this observation you will develop your own methods to facilitate this more easily, such as taking the respiratory rate whilst providing other personal care, washing or whilst in the vicinity of the patient.

Q) I find it difficult to co-ordinate counting the respirations whilst trying to monitor the time.

Many students find having to check their fob watch and count simultaneously difficult to do, as they miss the rise and fall of a patient's chest when they are monitoring the timing. You could place your

Table 7.5 **How to document a patient's respiratory rate**

Respirations per minute	01/09/20XX 08.00	Date/ Time	Date/ Time
> 30			
26–30			
21–25			
16–20			
11–15	13		
8–10			
< 8			

fob watch on the patient's bedside table (never on the bed) so that it is within your eye line and you can therefore concentrate solely upon counting the respiratory rate.

> *Note:* You should familiarize yourself with the correct technique and practise this skill before the OSCE, following the guidelines for measuring respiratory rate as described in this chapter.

Measuring, assessing and recording oxygen saturation measurement

Definition

Oxygen saturation is measured using a pulse oximeter. It is a common fallacy that a pulse oximeter indicates the level of oxygen in the blood. The majority of oxygen carried in the blood is bound to haemoglobin. Therefore having reduced haemoglobin level, as with anaemia, will result in less oxygen in the blood.

The pulse oximeter emits a red light which detects the colour difference between oxygenated and deoxygenated blood whilst identifying the pulse of the artery. It then uses this information to calculate the percentage of oxygen combined with haemoglobin. The measurement is always expressed as a percentage and the acceptable range is usually above 94% (BTS 2008). If the percentage rate indicated was less than 94% you would be expected to bring this to your mentor's attention and follow local policy guidelines.

Guidance for effective measurement of saturation

Always wash your hands and clean your equipment prior to commencing this skill. If there is a risk that your patient may have an infection or risk of personal contamination you should consider wearing gloves and apron, in accordance with local policy guidelines. Usually the oxygen saturation is measured by attaching the appropriate probe to either the patient's fingers, toes or ear lobes.

The pulse oximeter probe should be attached like a peg onto the patient's fingertip (see Fig. 7.5). You should be aware that the probe must be placed the correct way up; there may be a diagram on

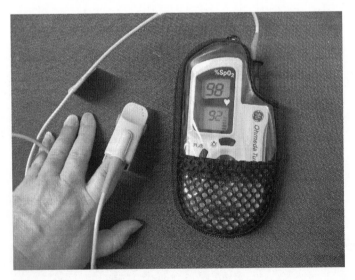

Figure 7.5 Using the pulse oximeter

the equipment to indicate this. You should ensure that the patient's selected finger is warm, has no nail varnish and they should be advised to keep their digit still whilst the measurement is being completed. Movement of the probe on the patient's finger, dirt or poor circulation will all affect the reading and could provide an inaccurate measurement. If the patient has symptoms of **shock** or trauma, peripheral shutdown may occur and this will reduce blood flow to the fingertips and other peripherals, therefore causing an inaccurate or unrecordable oxygen saturation reading. In peripheral vascular disease or diabetes blood flow may also be reduced to the peripheries.

Box 7.4 identifies normal ranges.

Box 7.4 Ranges for oxygen saturations

Measurements above 94% on room air are considered within normal range.

Documentation of oxygen saturation measurement

It is important to document your findings immediately after measuring the oxygen saturation, to ensure accuracy. Most clinical care settings will require the documentation to be completed using black ink. Your written documentation will be accessed by all members of the care team and may be utilized to inform patient treatment decisions; therefore it is imperative that your measurements cannot be misinterpreted.

Table 7.6 provides an example of how you would document a patient's oxygen saturation (SaO$_2$) that was found to be 96% on 2 L oxygen at 08.00 am. You should document the actual reading as a percentage on the chart, as well as indicating the flow rate or percentage of oxygen being administered. If a patient is not receiving additional oxygen you must still document their oxygen saturation, noting that the patient is breathing air. Prior to completing the OSCE you should familiarize yourself with the local documentation.

In this example the patient's oxygen saturation is within the acceptable range (indicated in white as between 96 and 100%). At this point the patient's oxygen saturation should not cause any concern. However, if a reading is found to be outside the acceptable range the student nurse would always be expected to bring this to their mentor's attention and follow local policy regarding actions that should be taken. In this case the patient's oxygen saturation level would be monitored as per their individual care pathway requirements.

Table 7.6 How to document a patient's oxygen saturation (SaO$_2$)

Oxygen saturation (%)	01/09/20XX 08.00	Date/ Time	Date/ Time
96–100	96%		
92–95			
85–91			
<85			
Litre/% oxygen	2 L		

Frequently asked question related to measuring oxygen saturations

Q) I have noticed that the pulse oximeter identifies the patient's pulse rate as well as their oxygen saturations. Is it alright for me to record the pulse rate for my OSCE assessment based on this reading, so that I do not have to manually assess the pulse?

No, the OSCE assessment requirements stipulate that you must be able to demonstrate your ability to manually assess the patient's pulse rate. Therefore your OSCE assessor is likely to ask you to measure the pulse manually prior to measuring the oxygen saturation.

Putting it all together!

The OSCE is likely to be performed in a clinical skills laboratory at your university campus, and you will generally have a time limit of between 20 and 30 minutes to complete all the observations. The room will be set up with a bed and a patient who could be either a manikin, a volunteer from outside the university, or a member of the wider teaching staff from your university school of nursing. In addition the room will have all the relevant equipment for you to carry out the procedures, such as thermometers and pulse oximeter.

Note: You should always ensure that your hands are clean prior to commencing the physical observation skills. This may be achieved by washing your hands using soap and water or by the application of cleansing hand gel, according to local policy.

The equipment must be cleaned using hard surface wipes before and after use on each individual patient according to local policy guidelines. Please ensure that the equipment has dried prior to use as damp equipment can encourage growth of microorganisms and will be uncomfortable for the patient.

You should approach the patient in a professional manner, providing an introduction including your name and role. You should also confirm how the patient would like to be addressed.

Prior to measuring the physical observations you should always gain the patient's consent by providing a clear explanation of what you are about to do and why the observations are required (NMC 2008).

You should identify if:

- The patient has rested for at least 5 minutes,
- They have eaten food or had any hot or cold fluid in the last 15 minutes,
- They have they been smoking.

Any of the above may create inaccuracy in your findings.

Box 7.5 **Putting it all together**

You will be expected to:
- Talk to the 'patient', gain their consent and ask any other relevant questions,
- Take the 'patient's' pulse, temperature, respiration rate and oxygen saturation.

Following the completion of the procedures you may be asked some questions about physiological measurements, so be prepared!

Having measured the physical observations (as outlined in the criteria in Table 7.7) the results should be accurately recorded using approved documentation. You will be assessed on your ability to accurately document your patient's physical observations as part of the OSCE.

 ## Examiners' marking criteria

Table 7.7 **Example of examiners' marking criteria**

Student's name and cohort year	
Expected performance criteria	Demonstrated Yes/No
All observations	
Student cleans hands (wash or alcohol gel).	
Student approaches patient in a professional manner with introduction.	
Student gains patient consent and co-operation and explains procedure to patient.	
Student reassures patient at the end of the procedures.	
Temperature	
Student ensures patient is in a comfortable position and has not eaten or drunk in the past 15 minutes.	
Student selects thermometer, either digital or tympanic (appropriate to patient's condition).	
Student ensures that thermometer has probe cover in place.	
Student places thermometer in appropriate site for appropriate amount of time.	
Student removes thermometer once electronic bleep audible.	
Student notes temperature and records accurately.	
Student removes probe and disposes of effectively.	
Student cleans equipment and returns to safe storage.	
Pulse and respirations	
Student ensures patient is in a comfortable position and has rested prior to taking pulse and respirations.	
Student ensures a clock or watch with second hand is easily visible.	
Student chooses an appropriate site for palpation.	
Student places second or third finger along the artery and presses gently.	

(continued)

Table 7.7 *(continued)*

Student's name and cohort year	
Expected performance criteria	Demonstrated Yes/No
Student counts and palpates the pulse for 60 seconds. Student also counts the respirations for an additional 60 seconds, whilst continuing to press on the radial artery, simultaneously assessing rhythm and depth.	
Student assesses patient's circulation.	
Student accurately records pulse and respiratory rates on the observation chart.	
Student is asked to comment upon rate, rhythm and amplitude of pulse.	
Student can answer questions related to temperature, pulse and respiration measurement.	

Examiners' questions

Note: Some universities may assess your knowledge in relation to physiological measurement and it is useful to prepare for that, if it is a requirement.

Example of typical questions an examiner may ask are provided in Box 7.6.

Box 7.6 **Example of examiners' questions**

1. Could you tell me the normal heart rate ranges?
2. Could you identify three normal sites for measuring pulse rates?
3. Could you identify three conditions where the heart rate may be high?
4. Could you identify three conditions where the heart rate may be low?
5. Could you explain the complications of tachycardia (at least two)?
6. Could you explain the complications of bradycardia (at least two)?
7. Could you explain when you would report an abnormal finding?
8. Could you tell me the normal respiratory rate (range)?
9. Could you describe the normal depth and rhythm of respiration?
10. Could you identify three conditions where the respiratory rate may be high?
11. Could you identify three conditions where the respiratory rate may be low?
12. Can you tell me normal oxygen saturation value?
13. When would you start saturation monitoring in practice?
14. Could you describe three situations when oxygen saturation may be abnormal?

15. Could you state three potential sources of error with oxygen saturation recording?
16. Could you explain when you would report abnormal findings?
17. Could you tell me the range for normal temperature?
18. Could you describe which sites can be used for temperature measurement and contraindications for each site?
19. Could you identify three conditions where the temperature may be high?
20. Could you identify three conditions where the temperature may be low?
21. Can you describe two complications of pyrexia?
22. Can you describe two complications of hypothermia?
23. Explain when you would report an abnormal finding?

Answers are provided at the end of the chapter.

✗ Common errors at this station

A number of errors occur at this station; these include failure to:

- Wash hands and decontaminate equipment prior to taking the observations,
- Place their fingers on the radial pulse site when taking the patient's pulse rate,
- Assess the strength and rhythm of the pulse as well as the rate,
- Use appropriate thermometer for type of patient,
- Ensure mode of tympanic thermometer is set correctly,
- Leave the thermometer in situ for the recommended time,
- Correctly position the pulse oximeter probe,
- Maintain communication with the patient throughout the OSCE,
- Document findings,
- Practise the correct technique before the OSCE.

✚ Top tips for passing this station

Ensure that you understand and follow any local guidelines and policies that relate to your OSCE.

- Make the most of any opportunities provided for practising the OSCE skills; this may be offered in clinical practice settings, as well as by the university lecturing team.
- Come to the OSCE dressed in appropriate uniform as per local guidelines.
- Maintain a professional attitude towards the 'patient' and the OSCE assessor.
- It is expected that you maintain communication with the 'patient' and assessor throughout the OSCE, including gaining consent, giving reassurance and providing an explanation of the readings obtained. Simply stating that an obtained result is fine does not demonstrate the required level of understanding the assessor is expecting to see.
- Ensure that the 'patient's' comfort is confirmed and maintained both during and after completion of the skill. You should provide an opportunity for the 'patient' to state if they found the assessment uncomfortable or too invasive.

- Always choose the equipment you are most familiar with.
- Try not to panic and keep calm.
- Remember, although the OSCE assessment is timed, you are permitted to reassess any one or more of the observations within the allotted time. This will allow you to confirm or retrieve any observations you may have experienced difficulty obtaining.
- It is good practice to always document each result as you go along; this will ensure that your documentation is accurate.

Please bear in mind, demonstrating ability to complete these skills is not just to enable you to pass the OSCE, but is a professional requirement as a practising registered nurse (NMC 2008). Therefore you will be expected to maintain the skills and associated knowledge throughout your nursing career.

 ## Online resource centre

You can find further advice and revision help for your OSCEs by going online now to see **www.oxfordtextbooks.co.uk/orc/caballero/**.

 ## References

British Thoracic Society (2008). *Guideline for Emergency Oxygen Use in Adult Patients*. London: British Thoracic Society.

Department of Health (2009). *Competencies for Recognising and Responding to Acutely ill Adults in Hospital. Draft guidelines for consultation*. London: Department of Health, HMSO.

Diggens, P. (2009). *Vital Signs*. In: Glasper, A., McEwing, G., Richardson, J. and Weaver M. (eds) *Foundation skills for caring, using student centred learning*. London: Palgrave MacMillan.

Marieb, E.N. and Hoehn, K. (2007). *Human Anatomy and Physiology*, 7th edn. San Francisco: Pearson Education.

National Institute of Health and Clinical Excellence (2007). *Acutely Ill Patients in Hospital: Recognition of and Response to Acute Illness of Adults in Hospital*. London: HMSO.

Nursing and Midwifery Council (2007). *Essential Skills Clusters (ESCs) for Pre-registration Nursing Programmes*. London: Nursing and Midwifery Council.

National Patient Safety Agency (2007). *Recognising and Responding Appropriately to Early Signs of Deterioration in Hospitalized Patients*. London: National Patient Safety Agency.

Nursing and Midwifery Council (2008). *The Code Standards of Conduct, Performance and Ethics for Nurses and Midwives*. London: Nursing and Midwifery Council.

 ## Appendix: answers to examiners' questions

1. Normal pulse range: 60–100 beats per minute (average 80 bpm).
   - Bradycardia: < 60 bpm,
   - Tachycardia: > 100 bpm.

2. Sites for pulse palpation: where artery travels over bone
   - Temporal,
   - Carotid,
   - Femoral,
   - Popliteal,
   - Posterior tibial,
   - Brachial,
   - Radial,
   - Dorsalis pedis,
   - Heart rate auscultation—apical/apex/apex-radial (atrial fibrillation).

3. Conditions where heart rate may be high:
   - Anxiety/sympathetic nervous system response,
   - Hyperthyroidism,
   - Shock (include all types),
   - Pyrexia,
   - Vasodilation,
   - Heart disease,
   - Incompatible blood transfusion,
   - Drug therapy,
   - Fluid loss/dehydration,
   - Pain.

4. Conditions where heart rate may be low:
   - Drugs—beta blockers,
   - Drugs, e.g. digoxin, amiodorone,
   - Athletes/physically fit,
   - Asleep,
   - Myxoedema,
   - Cardiac conduction problems,
   - Heart disease,
   - Cerebral bleeds (raised ICP).

5. Complications of tachycardia:
   - Reduced blood pressure as cardiac output reduced with reduced ventricular filling time,
   - Angina,
   - Myocardial infarction,
   - Syncope (fainting),
   - Increased O_2 requirement (increased respiratory rate).

6. Complications of bradycardia:
   - Reduced blood pressure as cardiac output = respiratory heart rate x stroke volume,
   - Dizziness,
   - Fainting.

7. Report when:
   - Overtly changed from baseline or patient's normal values,
   - > 100 bpm,
   - < 60 bpm,
   - Irregular/thready,
   - Patient unwell.

8. Normal respiratory rates (range): Male adult 14–18 breaths per minute, female adult 16–20 breaths per minute.

9. Depth: Tidal volume is approximately 500 ml/breath; use of spirometer to measure.
   Rhythm: Regular disorders in respiratory pattern often found in respiratory control centre disorders.
   Hyperventilation: increased rate and depth (exertion/fear/anxiety/fever/hepatic coma/midbrain and brainstem lesions/acid-base balance disturbance, e.g. diabetic ketoacidosis (DKA) or salicylate overdose—Kussmaul's respirations).
   > 20 bpm moderate, > 30 bpm severe
   Apneustic respirations = prolonged, gasping inspiration with short inefficient expiration (pons lesions).
   Cheyne-Stokes = periodic breathing
   Also, postoperative respirations/opiates/critically ill.

10. High respiratory rate: tachypnoea:
    - Extreme exertion,
    - Fear and anxiety,
    - Fever,

- Hepatic coma,
- Brainstem lesions,
- Acid-base balance disturbances, e.g. DKA/salicylate overdose,
- Alteration in blood gas concentrations,
- **Sepsis,**
- Chest or heart diseases in which pCO_2 rises or which cause hypoxia, e.g. COPD or pulmonary oedema.

11. Low respiratory rate: bradypnoea:
    - Respiratory depressants (drugs/opiates/anaesthesia),
    - Alcohol,
    - Sedation,
    - Brainstem lesions,
    - Head injury,
    - End of life (Cheyne-Stokes).

12. Normal oxygen saturation:
    - ≥ 94% and above, but seen in light of patient's medical history (e.g. COPD (Chronic obstructive pulmonary disease), respiratory history).

13. Indications for measuring oxygen saturation:
    - Monitoring oxygen therapy received,
    - During sedation/anaesthesia/mechanical ventilation,
    - Transport of the unwell patient/critically ill patient,
    - Haemodynamic instability: MI(myocardial infarction)/cardiac failure,
    - Assessment of respiratory illness/monitoring of same: COPD/asthma/bronchiectasis etc.
    - Any concerns over respiratory function or condition of the patient,
    - Monitoring during administration of respiratory depressant drugs, e.g. opiate epidurals/PCA (patient controlled analgesia),
    - Patient acutely unwell.

14. Situations when oxygen saturations may be abnormal:
    - Respiratory depression—drugs/head trauma/brainstem lesions,
    - Airways disease—asthma/bronchiectasis/COPD,
    - Acute changes in patient's condition: ill patient/sepsis,
    - Overdoses/anaesthetics/sedatives,
    - Carbon monoxide inhalation,
    - Hypoventilation,
    - Neuromuscular weakness, e.g. GBS (Gullian-Barre Syndrome), myasthenia gravis, etc.

15. Sources of error:
    - Nail varnish,
    - Dirt,
    - Foreign objects,
    - Bright or fluorescent room lighting,
    - Inappropriate probe, e.g. finger probe used on earlobe,
    - Movement—rigors/shivering,
    - Peripherally cold patient,
    - Peripheral vascular disease,
    - Low Hb.

16. Report:
    - Any concern about patient's condition,
    - Saturations which vary from patient's normal values.

17. Normal temperature range: 36–37°C (36–37.5°C in some texts).

18. Usual sites for temperature measurement:

- Oral/p.o. (contraindications: confused patient/ingestion of hot or cold fluid or food, oral surgery/mouth injuries/general anaesthesia),
- Rectal/p.r. (contraindications: rectal ulceration/perforation/soft stool/closed rectum),
- Axillary (contraindications: thin patient/confused patient),
- Tympanic (contraindications: positioning/hearing aids/tympanic membrane perforation/ear infection/ear wax).

19. Conditions where the temperature may be high: pyrexia/hyperthermia
    - Blood transfusion/blood products reaction,
    - Fever due to sepsis/infection/inflammation,
    - Hot environment: heat stroke/central heating/too many covers,
    - Neurological disturbance, e.g. damage to hypothalamus,
    - Post trauma,
    - Hyperthyroidism.

20. Conditions where the temperature may be low: hypothermia
    - Exposure/uncovered patient/damp patient,
    - Post surgery/general anaesthesia/cardiac surgery/neurosurgery,
    - Liver failure,
    - Hypothyroidism,
    - Cold infusions.

21. Complications of pyrexia:
    - Increased metabolic rate,
    - Increased oxygen requirements,
    - Seizures in children,
    - Discomfort,
    - Excess fluid loss (sweating),
    - Catabolic state.

22. Care includes:
    - Treat underlying condition (e.g. antibiotics for infection),
    - Antipyretics,
    - Tepid sponging,
    - Reducing environmental temperature,
    - Increasing nutrition if required,
    - Fanning may be mentioned,
    - Taking blankets off etc.

23. Complications of hypothermia:
    - Dysfunction of all organs especially central nervous and cardiovascular systems,
    - Listlessness,
    - Confusion,
    - Cardiac output initially rises with shivering, but then falls,
    - 28°C—spontaneous ventricular fibrillation,
    - Metabolism with falling temperature: increased blood glucose and increased potassium,
    - Kidneys cool—causes renal diuresis—hypovolaemia.

24. Care includes:
    - Passive warming: insulating blankets, hats,
    - Active warming: Bair Huggers,
    - Increasing environmental temperature,
    - Warming fluids,

25. Report any concern with temperature variation from patient's norm
    - Temperature > 37.5°C,
    - Temperature < 36°C.

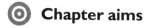

Chapter 8
Measuring blood pressure

Kate Devis

Chapter aims

This chapter will enable you to:

- Revise key material relating to this skill,
- Follow a step by step guide to taking blood pressure readings both manually and electronically,
- Understand how to prepare and revise for this OSCE,
- Highlight common problems at this station and how they may be avoided.

Introduction

Blood pressure measurements are one part of a circulatory assessment (Docherty and McCallum 2009). Treatments for raised or low blood pressure may be initiated or altered according to blood pressure readings; therefore correct measurement and interpretation of blood pressure is an important nursing skill.

Blood pressure should be determined using a standardized technique in order to avoid discrepancies in measurement (Torrance and Serginson 1996).

Both manual and automated **sphygmomanometers** may be used to monitor blood pressure. The manual auscultatory method of taking blood pressure is considered the gold standard (MRHA 2006), as automated monitoring can give false readings (Coe and Houghton 2002), and automated devices produced by different manufacturers may not give consistent figures (MRHA 2006). So, although automated sphygmomanometers are in common use within health care settings in the UK, the skill of taking blood pressure measurement manually is still required by nurses.

As a fundamental nursing skill, blood pressure measurement, using manual and automated sphygmomanometers, and interpretation of findings are often assessed via an OSCE.

Within this chapter revision of key areas will allow you to prepare thoroughly for your OSCE, in terms of practical skill and understanding of the procedure of taking blood pressure.

Key revision for your simulated examination

Systolic and diastolic values

Blood pressure is defined as the force exerted by blood against the walls of the vessels in which it is contained (Docherty and McCallum 2009). A blood pressure measurement uses two figures—the systolic and **diastolic** readings. The systolic reading is always the higher figure and represents the maximum pressure of blood against the artery wall during ventricular contraction. The diastolic reading represents the minimum pressure of the blood against the wall of the artery between ventricular contractions (Doughetry and Lister 2008). You will need to be able to accurately identify systolic and diastolic measurements during your OSCE.

Korotkoff's sounds

When a blood pressure cuff is applied to the upper arm and inflated above the level of systolic blood pressure no sounds will be detected when listening to the brachial artery with a stethoscope. The cuff clamps off blood supply. As the cuff is deflated a noise, which is usually a tapping sound, will be heard as the pressure equals the systolic blood pressure—this is the first **Korotkoff's sound.** It is important to listen carefully and note the reading on the sphygmomanometer when the first Korotkoff's sound is heard to ensure an accurate systolic reading.

As the cuff pressure is further released additional Korotkoff's sounds will be heard via the stethoscope, which are the noise of blood turbulence within the brachial artery (see Box 8.1). The sounds may be described as swishing and eventually become quite muffled. At the point when the sounds disappear completely the reading taken is the diastolic blood pressure. At this point the cuff no longer causes any resistance to blood flow. The Korotkoff's sound quality and type will not be identical for every person, which can be challenging for those learning how to measure blood pressure.

Recognition of hypotension and hypertension

Interpreting blood pressure measurements involves an understanding of normal values. In adults normal systolic blood pressure is within the range 100 to 139 millimetres of mercury (mmHg), and normal diastolic is between 60 and 90 mmHg (NICE/British Hypertensive Society 2006). It is important to be able to recognize any abnormalities in the blood pressure readings taken which are outside these ranges. There is no single normal blood pressure reading so it is important to compare findings with an individual's normal or baseline readings, to detect change or stability.

Hypertension, or high blood pressure, may be **chronic** or acute. NICE/British Hypertensive Society (2006) state that a constantly raised blood pressure above 140/90 mmHg is considered hypertension, and ongoing measurements of 160/100 mmHg require antihypertensive medications. Acute hypertension usually resolves once the cause has been addressed, e.g. this could be physical activity or anxiety.

Box 8.1 **The five phases of Korotkoff's sounds**

1. Faint but clear tapping sounds which increase gradually in intensity,
2. Softening of sounds which may become swishing,
3. The return of sharper sounds,
4. The distinct and abrupt muffling of sounds which become softer,
5. The point at which all sounds disappear.

Beevers et al. (2001)

Hypotension, or low blood pressure, is usually considered a symptom rather than a disease. Hypotension can be dangerous, particularly if diastolic pressure levels fall very low as then core body organs will not be well perfused with blood.

During the OSCE you will need to identify if the blood pressure measurements you take are normal, or if they indicate hypertension or hypotension.

Factors affecting blood pressure

A client's actual blood pressure, and therefore the reading taken, is affected by many factors. Some of these influences can be offset by a nurse's actions when taking non-urgent blood pressure measurements.

During an OSCE, as in practice, students should speak with the client and observe for signs of anxiety in recognition of 'white coat hypertension' (MRHA 2006). Speaking with the client and offering reassurance can help them relax. Nurses should also check if the client has been resting and if they are comfortable before taking measurements, as both exercise and pain can increase blood pressure (Tortora and Derrickson 2007). The client's physical position also influences blood pressure so nurses should check if previous measurements were taken in a lying or sitting position. Readings are lower when a client is seated (Neata *et al.* 2003).

Inaccuracies in measuring blood pressure

Inaccurate measurement of blood pressure has been attributed to several factors (a full list may be found in Box 8.2). Human error accounts for many inaccuracies so nurses should be aware of these factors in order to avoid them. Student nurses can perceive OSCE assessments as stressful and may consequently feel they will make a mistake, but practice and concentration can help minimize human error.

Box 8.2 Reasons for inaccurate blood pressure measurement

- Human (nurse) error:
  - Incorrect reading of the sphygmomanometer—unfamiliar with device,
  - Position of nurse when taking readings—unable to view manometer easily,
  - Lack of concentration,
  - Hearing problems,
  - Failure to interpret Korotkoff's sounds accurately,
  - Rounding off readings, e.g. commonly to zero, should not be done (e.g. 132/68 recorded as 130/70),
  - Observer prejudice, e.g. recording lower than measured figure for a young adult patient,
  - Failing to palpate for estimated blood pressure.
- Inappropriate cuff size for the client,
- Faulty or inadequately maintained equipment, e.g. leaking tubes or valves,
- Noisy workplace.

Alexis (2010); Beevers et al. (2001); MRHA (2006)

🖳 **Putting it all together!**

You may be given a choice of manual or automated sphygmomanometer to use when measuring blood pressure, or you may be advised which device to use. Listen carefully to the information you are given by the examiner as an introduction to the assessment. An automated adult skills model or an actor may be used to represent a client—in both situations the examiner will check the readings you take.

Ensure you use infection prevention strategies throughout the assessment. After you have received an introduction to the scenario remember to use appropriate hand hygiene before approaching the client. You should also clean equipment before use, particularly areas that may come into contact with the client including diaphragm and earpieces of the stethoscope and sphygmomanometer cuff. Alcohol/chlorhexadine wipes can be used to clean equipment as per local guidelines.

Step by step

Communication

- Consider the client's privacy.
- Explain the need to measure the client's blood pressure with him/her, discuss the procedure and check if consent is given.
- Ascertain how long the client has been resting in their current position. If the client has just been mobilizing or changed position advise the examiner and client that you will wait for 3 minutes before taking a reading.
- Check if any prior blood pressure measurements have been taken, and if so whether the client was seated or lying and which arm was used.
- Observe for any indicators which will allow you to determine which arm to use to take blood pressure measurements, e.g. the client may have an intravenous infusion running into one arm, or one arm may be oedematous or injured—so you would select the unaffected arm.
- Remember to continue to explain what you are doing to the client as you carry out the procedure.

Manual blood pressure measurement

Equipment

- Collect a stethoscope, sphygmomanometer with appropriate sized cuff and observation chart to ensure you are prepared properly.
- Check when the sphygmomanometer was last serviced and calibrated.
- Check the stethoscope chest piece is turned to amplify the diaphragm (plastic disc) rather than the bell side, and turn the earpieces so they fit comfortably. Position the stethoscope in your ears so that earpieces tilt forward. It is recommended that 'sounds are heard more clearly when the attachments follow the direction of the ear canal' (Kozier *et al.* 2008: 366).

Procedure

- Check that tight clothing is not constricting the client's arm.
- Apply the blood pressure cuff smoothly and firmly to the client's upper arm above the level of the brachial artery and in direct contact with skin.
- Check that the cuff bladder covers 80% of the arm circumference and that the cuff is aligned with the brachial artery, using the symbols or information on the cuff (sometimes an arrow; see Fig. 8.1a).

- The cuff should be positioned 2–3 cm above the **antecubital fossa.**
- Ask the client to rest their arm at heart level, and support their arm with a pillow if necessary.
- Palpate a radial pulse and inflate the cuff until this pulse can no longer be felt (see Fig. 8.1b).
- Empty the cuff of air and allow the client to rest for a minimum of 30 seconds.
- Palpate for the **brachial pulse** (see Fig. 8.1c) and place the diaphragm of the stethoscope directly where the brachial pulse was palpated. The stethoscope should not be tucked under the cuff.
- Inflate the cuff to 30 mmHg above the radial pulse reading for systolic pressure (Dougherty and Lister 2008).
- Deflate the cuff slowly at a rate of 2 mmHg per second whilst listening for Korotkoff's sounds (see Fig. 8.1d).
- Take care to avoid leaving the cuff inflated for prolonged periods as this will cause significant discomfort to your patient.
- Note the systolic and diastolic blood pressures and then completely deflate the cuff.
- If you have not heard either or both pressures correctly then allow the patient to rest for 3 minutes and repeat the procedure.

Post procedure

- Ensure the client is left in a comfortable position and offer them information on your findings.
- Clean equipment as appropriate, and then wash your hands.
- Record your measurements by documenting accurately on the observation chart and be prepared to discuss interpretation of findings with the examiner.
- You should look for any baseline reading with which to compare your measurement.

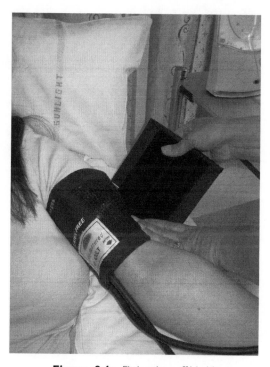

Figure. 8.1a Fitting the cuff bladder

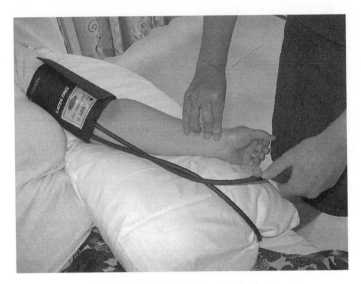

Figure 8.1b Palpate the radial pulse

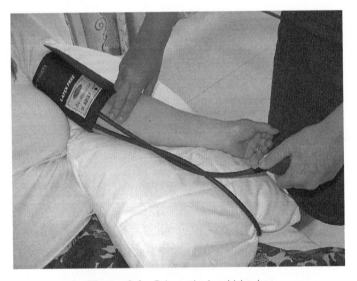

Figure 8.1c Palpate the brachial pulse

Automated blood pressure measurement: step by step guide

Equipment

- Collect an automated sphygmomanometer.
- Check when it was last serviced and calibrated.
- If necessary change the cuff to one of an appropriate size for the client you have been asked to assess.
- Ensure you also have an observation chart to record your findings.

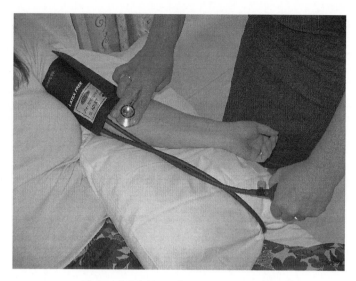

Figure 8.1d Listen for Korotkoff's sounds

Procedure

- Check pulse rhythm at the radial artery. If arrhythmias are present inform the examiner as this can cause an inaccurate reading when using an automated sphygmomanometer.
- Switch the sphygmomanometer on and check the display panel illuminates.
- Ask the client to rest their arm at heart level, and support with a pillow if appropriate.
- Apply cuff smoothly and firmly to the client's upper arm so it fits snugly above the level of the brachial artery and is in direct contact with skin. Some automated devices require positioning of the cuff bladder over the brachial artery so ensure cuff is correctly in place.
- Advise the patient to keep still whilst the machine is working.
- Press the button to inflate the cuff.
- Once the device has taken the reading note systolic and diastolic pressures.
- If a repeat reading is required wait at least 1 minute before re-inflating the cuff.

Post procedure

- Remove the cuff promptly and ensure the client is left feeling comfortable.
- Offer the client information on your findings.
- Clean equipment as appropriate, ensure automated device is left plugged in to charge, and then wash your hands.
- Record your measurements accurately on the observation chart and be prepared to discuss interpretation of findings with the examiner.
- You should look for any baseline reading with which to compare your measurement.

Recording blood pressure measurements

- The systolic and diastolic pressures should be recorded as a double-ended arrow on the appropriate section of the observation chart.
- It is not necessary to add the figures, as the points of each arrow will indicate them. In addition, using only arrows allows trends in blood pressure to be easily visualized.

Examiners' marking criteria

Table 8.1 **Example of examiners' marking criteria**

Student's name and cohort year	
Expected performance criteria	Demonstrated Yes/No
<ul><li>Student cleans hands,</li><li>Student approaches patient in a professional manner and introduces self,</li><li>Student explains the need for recording blood pressure in terms the patient can understand,</li><li>Student explains the procedure to the patient and gains consent,</li><li>Student ensures the patient is in a comfortable position and has rested for at least 3 minutes,</li><li>The patient's arm is positioned correctly (level with heart, clothing removed to facilitate procedure),</li><li>The student estimates the systolic pressure by initially inflating cuff until radial pulse can no longer be felt, and informs the assessor of the estimated reading,</li><li>The cuff is deflated and student waits 30 seconds until re-inflating,</li><li>The patient's comfort is checked and the patient is observed,</li><li>The cuff is inflated again to 30 mmHg higher than estimated systolic pressure,</li><li>The diaphragm of the stethoscope is placed over the brachial artery in correct position,</li><li>The systolic pressure is recorded at the correct time,</li><li>The diastolic pressure is recorded at the correct time,</li><li>The measurement is accurately documented,</li><li>The student ensures the patient is left in a comfortable position,</li><li>Student cleans hands.</li></ul>	

Examiners' questions

You may be asked questions to assess your knowledge underpinning blood pressure measurement. Possible questions are provided in Box 8.3.

Box 8.3 **Example of examiners' questions**

1. What is the normal range for blood pressure in adults?
2. What does systolic pressure represent?
3. What does diastolic pressure represent?
4. Can you identify three conditions where the blood pressure may be high?
5. Can you identify three conditions where the blood pressure may be low?

6. What are two of the complications of hypotension?

7. What are two of the complications of hypertension?

8. Explain when you would report an abnormal finding.

9. How do you decide which cuff is the correct size for this patient?

10. How do you decide where to place the cuff?

Answers are provided at the end of the chapter.

✗ Common errors at this station

As measuring blood pressure involves a number of important steps, and measurement using a manual sphygmomanometer involves technical skill, there are numerous possible problems that students may experience. The following section provides extra tips, but these are some of the common mistakes students may make:

- Not cleaning hands before approaching the client,
- Forgetting to estimate the systolic pressure using radial pulse occlusion, before listening for blood pressure,
- Not cleaning equipment before and after using with the client,
- Not fitting cuff snugly enough or placing it too low on the client's arm,
- Forgetting to palpate the brachial artery,
- Not knowing the anatomical position of brachial artery,
- Putting the stethoscope in wrong position,
- Not identifying Korotkoff's sounds correctly and so making inaccurate readings,
- Falsifying readings as cannot hear Korotkoff's sounds adequately,
- Not taking client's comfort into account, e.g. leaving their arm suspended in mid-air,
- Leaving the cuff inflated for far too long, so that, e.g., the client's fingers begin to turn blue,
- Not using hand hygiene after patient contact,
- Not documenting results accurately,
- Stethoscope not placed correctly in ears,
- Misreading the figures on the dial—some are marked in single digits and some in twos.

✚ Top tips for passing this station

These are some suggestions to help you prepare and pass this station, based on experience assessing students taking blood pressure measurements during OSCE.

- It can be difficult to remember the client when you are trying hard to remember the procedure, but do speak to the client when you are taking blood pressure measurements and check their comfort.
- Make sure you position the cuff high enough up the client's upper arm, so that it will not cover the diaphragm of the stethoscope when in position.
- It is not possible to hear Korotkoff's sounds, and therefore blood pressure, if the stethoscope is not correctly located. Always palpate for brachial pulse before placing the diaphragm of the stethoscope in position.

- Use your dominant hand for pumping up and deflating the cuff—this will allow you more control so you can deflate the cuff steadily.
- Do not deflate the cuff too quickly—a steady pace of 2 mmHg a second will allow you to take accurate readings.
- If you have not been able to hear the Korotkoff's sounds or you are unsure about the readings, advise the client and the examiner that you will need to retake the blood pressure measurements. For safety reasons it is always best to be honest if you are unsure. If you are confident you have accurately estimated the systolic blood pressure using radial pulse occlusion you will not need to repeat this step.
- Infection prevention is important—remember to clean your hands and your equipment before and after use.

 ## Online resource centre

You can find further advice and revision help for your OSCEs including a video of measuring blood pressure by going online now to see **www.oxfordtextbooks.co.uk/orc/caballero/**.

 ## References

Alexsis, O. (2010). Providing best practice in manual blood pressure measurement. *British Journal of Nursing,* 18(7): 410–415.

Beevers, G. *et al.* (2001). Blood pressure measurement. *British Medical Journal,* 322: 1043–1047.

Coe, T. and Houghton, K. (2002). Comparison of the automated Dinamap blood pressure monitor with the mercury sphygmomanometer for detecting hypertension in the day case pre-assessment clinic. *Journal of Ambulatory Surgery,* 10: 9–15.

Docherty, C. and McCallum, J. (eds) (2009). *Foundation Clinical Nursing Skills.* Oxford: Oxford University Press.

Dougherty, L. and Lister, L. (2008). *The Royal Marsden Manual of Clinical Nursing Procedures,* 7th edn. Chichester: John Wiley & Sons.

Kozier, B., Erb, G., Berman, A., Snyder, S., Lake, R. and Harvey, S. (2008). Fundamentals of nursing, concepts, process and practice. Harlow: Pearson Education.

MRHA (2006). Device Bulletin—Blood Pressure Measurement Devices DB2006(03) [Published online]. http://www.mhra.gov.uk/Publications/Safetyguidance/DeviceBulletins/CON2024245.

Neata, R. *et al.* (2003). Both arm and body position significantly influence blood pressure measurement. *Journal of Human Hypertension,* 17: 459–462.

NICE/British Hypertensive Society (2006). *NICE Clinical Guideline 34. Hypertension: management of hypertension in adults in primary care* [Published online]. http://www.nice.org.uk/nicemedia/live/10986/30114/30114.pdf.

Torrance, C. and Serginson, E. (1996). Student nurses' knowledge in relation to blood pressure measurement by sphygmomanometery and auscultation. *Nurse Education Today,* 16: 397–402.

Tortora, G. and Derrickson, B. (2007). *Principles of Anatomy and Physiology* 12th edn. New York: John Wiley & Sons.

 ## Appendix: answers to examiners' questions

1. What is the normal range for blood pressure in adults?
   100/60 mmHg–140/90 mmHg
   Hypertension: systolic blood pressure ≥ 140 mmHg and diastolic blood pressure > 90 mmHg
   Hypotension: systolic blood pressure < 100 mmHg

2. What does systolic blood pressure represent?
   It is the peak pressure of blood against arterial walls caused by ventricular contraction.

3. What does diastolic blood pressure represent?
   It is the minimum pressure of blood against arterial walls following closure of aortic valve.

4. Can you identify three conditions where the blood pressure may be high?
   Select from:
   - Arteriosclerosis,
   - Familial hypertension,
   - Stress/anxiety/sympathetic nervous system response,
   - Thyrotoxicosis,
   - Fever,
   - Physical exertion,
   - Obesity,
   - Retention of sodium and water,
   - Increased fluid volume,
   - Vasoconstriction,
   - Pregnancy,
   - Renal problems,
   - Cerebral haemorrhage,
   - Pain,
   - High caffeine intake,
   - History of smoking.

5. Can you identify three conditions where the blood pressure may be low?
   Select from:
   - Postural hypotension,
   - Shock—including cardiogenic/septic/hypovolaemic/anaphylaxis/toxic shock syndrome,
   - Fluid/plasma loss—vomiting/diarrhoea/dehydration/burns,
   - Cardiac drugs—antihypertensives, beta blockers, ace inhibitors,
   - Opiate drugs,
   - Spinal blockade/epidural,
   - Bradycardia,
   - Tachycardia,
   - Cardiac damage,
   - Vasodilatation.

6. What are two of the complications of hypotension?
   These include:
   - Reduced tissue/organ perfusion,
   - Reduced mean arterial pressure (MAP),
   - Fainting/syncope/light-headedness/pallor/pre-renal failure,
   - Decreased urine output.

7. What are two of the complications of hypertension?
   These include:
   - Renal damage,
   - Headaches,
   - Visual disturbance,
   - Vessel damage,
   - Myocardial infarction,
   - Cerebrovascular accident,
   - Embolism,
   - Aneurysms.

8. Explain when you would report an abnormal finding.

    Report when one or more of the following occur:

    - Deviation from normal values for patient,
    - When indicated by MEWS or observations,
    - Any concern about the patient,
    - If the patient appears unwell.

9. The cuff should be able to cover 80% of the circumference of the upper arm.

10. Assess whether any of the limbs are inappropriate for the recording of blood pressure (such as intravenous infusion site).

    - Place the cuff 2–3 cm above the antecubital fossa,
    - Ensure that the cuff is aligned with the brachial artery, using the symbols or information on the cuff (sometimes an arrow).

Chapter 9
Urinalysis

Jane Lovegrove

Chapter aims

This chapter will enable you to:

- Revise key material relating to this skill,
- Follow a step by step guide to performing both **macroscopic** and chemical analysis,
- Understand how to prepare and revise for this OSCE,
- Highlight common problems at this station and how they may be avoided.

Introduction

Urinalysis simply means analysis of urine. It is an easily performed investigation that can detect a wide variety of abnormalities within a few minutes at low cost. Urinalysis is an investigation which all nurses should be competent to perform and is identified by the NMC (2007) as being an example of an essential skill nurse students should be competent to perform before entering their branch programme.

Urinalysis may be performed in a wide variety of clinical settings. It should be performed on every patient entering the acute care setting. Additionally, the National Confidential Enquiry into Patient Outcome and Death (NCEPOD (2009), stresses the need for urinalysis to be performed on all emergency admissions to an acute hospital. It may also be performed in outpatient and general practice clinics, and community areas.

To obtain the most accurate information from the test, students need to know how to obtain and assess a sample of urine and be aware of factors that may influence the reliability of the investigation.

Key revision for your simulated examination

Urine may be tested in three different ways:

- Macroscopic urinalysis,
- Microscopic urinalysis,
- Chemical analysis.

Macroscopic and chemical analysis are the investigations performed in the clinical setting which may be tested by OSCE. Microscopic investigation requires samples to be sent to a laboratory. Macroscopic analysis is the analysis of the urine by the naked eye. Chemical analysis may be performed by use of a plastic diagnostic **reagent strip** or 'dipstick' which contains small pads of chemicals which react to substances that may be found in urine.

Obtaining a sample of urine

For purposes of testing urine at random, clients are asked to urinate into a clean but not sterile dry container with no precautions regarding contamination. In females in particular this may result in samples being contaminated by vaginal fluids, such as blood or mucus. Due to the risk of contamination a mid-stream specimen of urine may be required if an abnormality is found in a random sample. A mid-stream specimen requires cleaning of the external urethral meatus prior to urination, passing the first half of the bladder contents into the lavatory, and passing the second part of the urine flow into a sterile container. The second half of the urine flow is then used for analysis. This method is also used to obtain a sample for **microscopic analysis** in the laboratory. Having obtained the sample it should be tested as soon as possible, and within 2 hours of obtaining the sample (Siemens Healthcare Diagnostics 2008).

Macroscopic urinalysis

The appearance of urine is examined by visual inspection. Normal urine is pale to dark yellow in colour and clear. Any cloudiness or debris in the urine should be noted together with any change in colour. Cloudiness may be caused by cell debris, or may be due to infection. Red brown urine may be caused by eating beetroot, drugs or the presence of red blood cells, haemoglobin or myoglobin, a pigment found in muscle. Very yellow/orange urine may be due to the presence of urobilinogen or drugs such as Rifampicin. Changes in urine colour need to be reported as some causes may result in damage to tissue. Haemaoglobin and myoglobin may block renal tubules. Infected urine may smell of fish. Urine that has stood for some time may smell of ammonia. Normally urine should not smell.

Chemical analysis

Routine chemical analysis may be performed with the use of a diagnostic reagent strip of a variety of substances, the range of which varies according to which type of strip is selected. The most commonly used tests are listed here:

- pH,
- Specific gravity,
- Protein,
- Glucose,
- Ketones,
- Blood haemolysed and non-haemolysed,
- Nitrates,
- Urobilinogen,
- Bilirubin.

pH

Normal range—4.5 to 8.0

The pH scale measures the hydrogen ion concentration. Urine pH is normally found to range from 7.4 to 6; however, depending on the acid base status, urinary pH may range from as low as 4.5 acid urine, to 8.0 alkali urine. The pH of the blood should be 7.35—7.45; to maintain this, the kidneys in health are able to excrete excess acid or alkali ingested or created, which then appears in the urine.

Specific gravity

Normal range—1.001 to 1.035

Specific gravity measures urine density, that is the concentration of solute within the urine. Low specific gravity indicates dilute urine with low solute concentrations. This may be as a result of use of diuretics, but may indicate renal impairment or diabetes insipidus. High specific gravity indicates concentrated urine usually due to dehydration, but may indicate high levels of glucose or presence of other contaminants.

Glucose

Normal range—negative

Urine should not contain glucose. While glucose does pass through the glomerulus it should all be reabsorbed in the proximal convoluted tubule. However, glucose will appear in urine if the blood glucose level rises.

Protein

Normal range—negative

Urine should not normally contain protein. Small amounts of protein may be filtered by the glomerulus but all should be reabsorbed by the renal tubules. Protein may be found due to contamination of urine by mucus. Protein may also be due to infection, presence of blood or glomerular damage. If protein is found when testing a random sample, a mid-stream specimen should be requested; if this is also positive to protein further investigation is required.

Blood—non-haemolysed

Normal range—negative

Normally no blood is detectable in urine. Normal red blood cells are too large to pass through the glomerulus. If non-haemolysed blood is present in urine it may have entered the urinary tract after the glomerulus as a result of urinary stones or trauma of the urinary tract. Other causes are glomerular damage or kidney trauma. Red blood cells may also contaminate urine from the vagina in menstruating women.

Blood—haemolysed

Normal value—negative

As previously stated normal red blood cells are too large to pass through the glomerulus. However, haemoglobin may be released from red blood cells when damaged as free haemoglobin and this may pass through the glomerulus and enter the urine. Urine positive to haemolysed blood requires further investigation.

Bilirubin

Normal value—negative

Bilirubin is formed from the breakdown of haemoglobin. Excess bilirubin may be formed due to excessive breakdown of red cells, e.g. following large blood transfusion. High blood levels of bilirubin may also occur as a result of liver disease or bile duct obstruction. Reagent strips measure conjugated bilirubin. Conjugated bilirubin is water soluble bilirubin which is normally excreted into the bowel and converted to urobilinogen by intestinal bacteria, giving faeces their brown colour. Bilirubin in the urine is abnormal and may indicate liver disease or biliary disease.

Urobilinogen

Normal range—trace

Urobilinogen is formed in the gut by breakdown of conjugated bilirubin by intestinal bacteria. Urobilinogen is normally excreted in faeces but small amounts may be reabsorbed and excreted in urine. Small amounts of urobilinogen are normally present in urine.

Large amounts of urobilinogen may occur in hepatic disease or excessive breakdown of red blood cells.

Ketones

Normal value—negative

Ketones which comprise acetone, acetoacetic acid and beta-hydroxybutyric acid are produced from the burning of fat to produce energy. Ketones may be present in urine resulting from diabetes mellitus or starvation. If ketones are found then blood glucose should also be tested.

Nitrite

Normal value—negative

A positive nitrite test indicates bacteria may be present in the urine in significant numbers. Nitrite is created by the conversion of nitrate from the diet to nitrite by Gram negative bacteria. Where urine is positive to nitrite, a mid-stream specimen of urine should be sent to the laboratory for culture and sensitivity.

Leucocytes

Normal range—negative

A positive result test results from the presence of white blood cells which may be whole white cells or lysed white cells. A positive test indicates infection and requires further investigation using a mid-stream specimen of urine. A negative test indicates that infection is unlikely and that without further evidence of infection there is no requirement for further investigation.

Putting it all together!

An overview of urinalysis procedure can be seen in Box 9.1.

> **Box 9.1 Putting it all together!**
>
> 1. Urine is a body fluid and universal precautions should be taken. Put on a plastic apron and clean gloves (see Fig. 9.1a).
> 2. Collect a fresh urine sample—note for the purpose of OSCEs samples are generally provided (see Fig. 9.1b).
> 3. Check expiry dates of diagnostic reagent strips (see Fig. 9.1c).

4. Dip all the test pads of the reagent strip into the urine and remove immediately (see Fig. 9.1d).

5. Drag the edge of the strip against the container rim to remove excess urine (see Fig. 9.1e).

6. Read each pad at the designated time shown on the side of the bottle containing the reagent strips (see Fig. 9.1f).

7. Dispose of reagent strip in appropriate waste bin.

8. Remove gloves and record results (see Fig. 9.1g).

9. Remove apron (see Fig. 9.1h).

10. Wash hands using soap and water (see Fig. 9.1i)

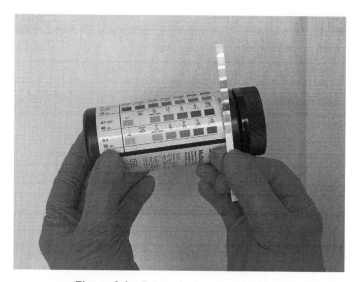

Figure 9.1a Put on plastic apron and gloves

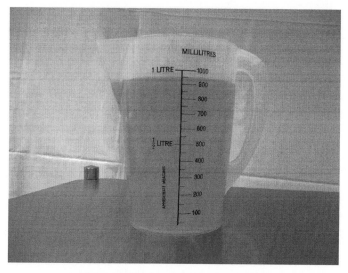

Figure 9.1b Collect fresh urine sample

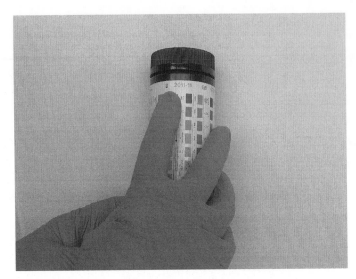

Figure 9.1c Check expiry dates on diagnostic reagent strips

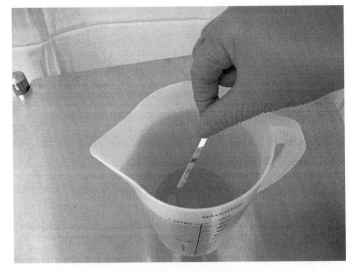

Figure 9.1d Dip test pads into urine

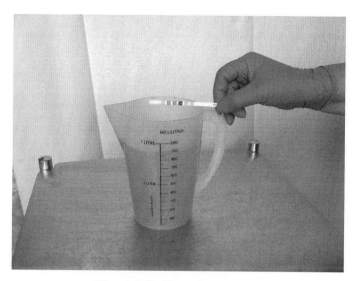

Figure 9.1e Remove excess urine

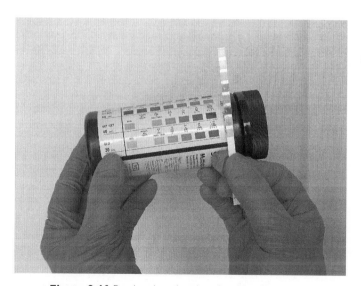

Figure 9.1f Read each pad against the side of the bottle

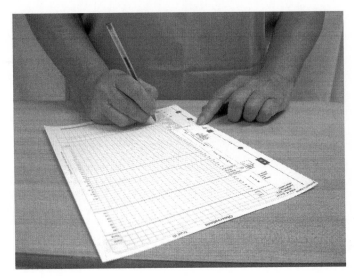

Figure 9.1g Record results

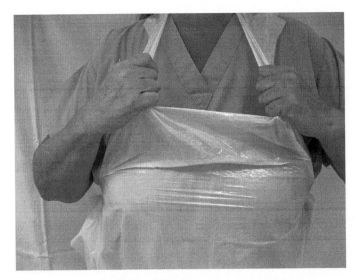

Figure 9.1h Remove apron

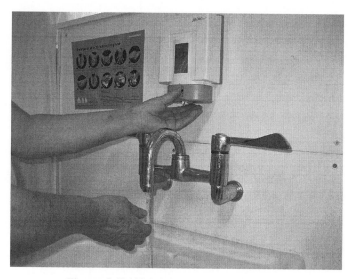

Figure 9.1i Wash hands using soap and water

✓ Examiners' marking criteria

Various tools will be utilized to assess your competence when performing urinalysis. As stated in earlier chapters it is advisable to review your own university's marking criteria. An example of marking criteria is included in Table 9.1.

Table 9.1 **Example of examiners' marking criteria**

Student's name and cohort year	
Expected performance criteria	Demonstrated Yes/No
Student complies with infection control dress code policy—hair is off the collar, short sleeves, no wrist watches and only one plain wedding band where institutional policy allows. Some settings may not require uniform.	
Student cleans hands by either hand wash or alcohol gel.	
Student puts on apron and clean non-sterile gloves.	
Student obtains specimen of urine in clean dry container (normally provided for OSCE purposes).	
Student checks expiry date of diagnostic reagent strips.	
Student removes one reagent strip from the bottle and reseals the bottle.	
Student dips all pads on the reagent strip into the urine and removes immediately.	

(continued)

Table 9.1 (*continued*)

Student's name and cohort year	
Expected performance criteria	Demonstrated Yes/No
Student drags the edge of the reagent strip on the rim of the container to remove excess urine.	
Student compares each test pad to the colour blocks on the bottle label at the indicated time, taking care not to contaminate the bottle.	
Student discards reagent strip into clinical waste bin.	
Student removes gloves and discards into clinical waste bin.	
Student records results.	
Student removes apron.	
Student washes hands.	
Student copies results on to clean paper that may be taken into clinical area.	

Examiners' questions

You may be asked questions to assess your knowledge underpinning urinalysis. Possible questions are outlined in Box 9.2.

Box 9.2 **Example of examiners' questions**

1. Name three normal constituents of urine.
2. What is the pH range of normal urine?
3. What does specific gravity measure?
4. What is the normal range of specific gravity for urine?
5. What would a specific gravity of 1.003 indicate?
6. What would a specific gravity of 1.030 indicate?
7. If glucose is found in the urine what action should be taken?
8. If ketones are found in the urine what action should be taken?
9. State two reasons why ketones may be found in urine.
10. What does the pH scale measure?
11. When may bilirubin be found in urine?
12. What is urobilinogen?
13. What does the presence of nitrites in the urine indicate?
14. What action should be taken if the test for leucocytes is positive?
15. What is the difference between non-haemolysed and haemolysed blood?

Answers are provided at the end of the chapter.

Common errors at this station

A number of errors can occur at this station and these include:

- Failure to wear an apron,
- Failure to check expiry date of reagent strips.

Very common errors include:

- Leaving the reagent strip in the urine too long,
- Failure to time readings of reagent pads,
- Contamination of watch by handling with gloved hand which previously held reagent strip,
- Contamination of pen by handling with gloved hand,
- Failure to record pH and specific gravity,
- Forgetting results.

 Top tips for passing this station

- Urine is a body fluid, so gloves and apron must be worn when performing urinalysis.
- A fresh sample of urine is required. Samples over 2 hours old should be discarded.
- Urinalysis reagent strips should be stored as directed by the manufacturer and not used after the expiry date.
- Reagent strips should not be held in urine but removed immediately once pads are covered in urine.
- Reagent strips should be held horizontally to prevent fluid from one pad running into another.
- Reagent pads must be read at time specified.
- To avoid cross infection. watches and pens should not be handled with a gloved hand that has held a reagent strip or reagent strip bottle.
- A value must be entered when recording results for pH and specific gravity.
- Paper that has been placed on a sluice surface to record results should not be taken into the clinical area.

 Online resource centre

You can find further advice and revision help for your OSCEs by going online now to see www.oxfordtextbooks.co.uk/orc/caballero/.

References

NCEPOD (2009) *Adding Insult to Injury: A Review of the Care of Patients Who Died in Hospital with a Primary Diagnosis of Acute Kidney Injury.* . London: NCEPOD.
Nursing and Midwifery Council (2007). *Essential Skills Clusters.* London: Nursing and Midwifery Council.
Siemens Healthcare Diagnostics (2008). Data sheet for diagnostics reagent strips for urinalysis. Dcerfield, Ille Siemens.

Appendix: answers to examiners' questions

1. Answer could include water, urea, creatinine and sodium potassium among others.

2. The range of pH is 4.6–8.0.

3. Specific gravity measures the density of the urine, the water to solute ratio.

4. The range of specific gravity for urine is 1.001 to 1.035.

5. A specific gravity of 1.003 indicates dilute urine; this may be due to excessive fluid intake, diuretics or diabetes insipidus.

6. A specific gravity of 1.030 indicates concentrated urine. This may be due to dehydration, reduced fluid intake, high glucose levels or contamination by substances such as radio opaque dyes.

7. If glucose is found in the urine, blood glucose should also be taken.

8. If ketones are found in the urine, investigations should be made to establish whether the person is in a state of starvation or has diabetes mellitus. Blood glucose should be tested.

9. Ketones are found in urine due to the metabolism of fat to provide energy; this may be due to starvation or diabetes mellitus.

10. The pH scale measures the hydrogen ion concentration, the degree of acidity or alkalinity.

11. Bilirubin may be found in urine in liver disease.

12. Urobilinogen is derived from bilirubin which is converted to urobilinogen by bacteria in the gut. Urobilinogen gives faeces their yellow brown colour.

13. Nitrite in the urine indicates the presence of bacteria. Nitrates derived from the diet are converted into nitrite by the bacteria.

14. Leucocytes indicate the presence of whole or lysed white blood cells. Therefore a specimen should be sent to the laboratory for testing.

15. Non-haemolysed blood is whole red blood cells; these are too large to pass through the glomerulus in normal circumstances. Haemolysed blood is lysed red blood cells which release their haemoglobin. Haemoglobin is small enough to pass through the glomerulus.

Chapter 10
Assessment of medication calculation skills

Terry Stubbings

 Chapter aims

This chapter will enable you to:

- Revise key material relating to this skill,
- Understand how to prepare and revise for this OSCE by providing opportunities to calculate medication.

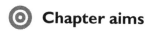 **Introduction**

Accuracy with medication dosage calculation is key to safe practice for a nurse. However, errors are not uncommon and seem to be increasing in frequency and some of them lead to harm or death to patients (NPSA 2009).

The NMC (2010), in its essential skills clusters, requires baseline skills for calculating medicines, nutrition and fluids. It also requires that, by completion of a nursing course, an individual will be competent in the process of medication related calculation involving tablets and capsules, liquid medicines, injections and IV infusions. Part of this competence is making judgements about what calculations to use, how to do them, what degree of accuracy is appropriate and what the answer means in relation to the context.

Passing an assessment of medication dosage calculation skills should be seen as only one aspect of developing the competence to practise safely.

Your medication dosage calculation assessment

There are three possible approaches to assessment on nursing courses:

Practice based assessment   If this is how medication related calculation skills are assessed on your course, you should feel confident that it has a high degree of validity (that is, the assessment is very real, since it is done in a real clinical environment). However, the many variables in a clinical setting mean that the assessment can be considered low in reliability (that is, that the same level of medication related calculation skill would be assessed each time). If your course requires this sort of assessment, ensure you find out exactly what is being assessed. Is the assessment just about calculation of medication dosages, or are other aspects of medication administration also being tested (e.g. assessment of patient prior to administration, interpersonal skills with patients, administration, documentation)? Documentation of medication administered is very important in nursing practice, so this aspect is likely to be included.

Objective structured clinical examination (OSCE) If this is how medication related calculation skills are assessed on your course, you should feel confident that it has a high degree of reliability (that is, assessment can be carried out in the same way with each student) and the level of validity is quite high too (that is, it will be set up like a real clinical environment).

  If your course requires this sort of assessment, ensure you find out exactly what is being assessed. Some universities include a medication dosage calculation element within an ALS or Trauma OSCE. You need to be sure if the assessment is just about calculation of medication dosages, or are other aspects of medication administration also being tested (e.g. interpersonal skills with a mock patient, administration, documentation)?

A computer based assessment process If this is how medication related calculation skills are assessed on your course, you should feel confident that it has a high degree of reliability and validity (as shown by Hutton *et al.* 2010). Many nursing courses utilize computer programs such as that supplied by Authentic World®. If your course requires this sort of assessment, ensure you take opportunities to familiarize yourself with the software, as well as practising calculation of medication dosages.

  For any type of assessment you need to know whether calculators and/or written formulae and/or paper and pen can be used during the assessment.

  Don't forget that clinical areas are ideal for practising medication dosage calculation since the context in which calculations are performed contributes to accuracy (Jukes and Gilchrist 2006), so practice in a wide range of clinical settings would be helpful.

  The increasingly technological nature of nursing means that calculators are a useful tool to reduce arithmetical errors, but if you rely on one, you must ensure that you know exactly what calculations you are attempting, since many errors in nursing calculations are conceptual errors (Sabin 2001).

Key revision for your simulated examination

The metric system and SI units

In 1960 there was widespread international agreement to adopt a system of metric weights and measures and British health care settings generally follow this Système International (SI). Unfortunately the USA has not adopted such SI units and therefore they are not used in many American textbooks.

  The SI system is a metric system. When it comes to medication there are only two units that you need to know: the unit of mass (weight) which is the gram (g) and the unit of volume which is the litre (l).

Multiples of units or fractions of units are expressed through prefixes

You also need to know the prefix milli, which means *one thousandth of* and micro which means *one millionth of,* i.e.

- 1 milligram (mg) is a thousandth of a gram (g). There are 1,000 milligrams in a gram.
- 1 microgram (sometimes abbreviated to mcg but ideally written in full) is a millionth of a gram (g). There are 1,000,000 micrograms in a gram.

- 1 microgram (mcg) is a thousandth of a milligram (mg). There are 1,000 micrograms in a milligram.
- 1 millilitre (ml) is a thousandth of a litre (l). There are 1,000 millilitres in a litre.

Because the metric system is all about tens, hundreds, thousands etc. and about tenths, hundredths, thousandths etc.,converting one set of units to another is all about multiplying or dividing by ten, a hundred, a thousand etc.

Converting

This can be done by *moving the decimal point.*

To multiply by 10 move the decimal point 1 place to the right (e.g. 0.15 × 10 = 01.5).

To multiply by 100 move the decimal point 2 places to the right (e.g. 0.15 × 100 = 15).

To multiply by 1,000 move the decimal point 3 places to the right (e.g. 0.15 × 1,000 = 150).

To divide by 10 move the decimal point 1 place to the left. (e.g. 0.15 ÷ 10 = 0.015).

To divide by 100 move the decimal point 2 places to the left. (e.g. 0.15 – 100 = 0.0015).

To divide by 1,000 move the decimal point 3 places to the left (e.g. 0.15 ÷1,000 = 0.00015).

In conversions related to medication, you will usually be dividing or multiplying by 1,000 (moving decimal point 3 places, left or right).

> Note: What if there isn't a decimal point in the number? It doesn't matter because any whole number can be thought of as that number, *point zero*, e.g. 500 = 500.0.

And by adding a decimal point at the end of the whole number you will have a decimal point to move.

In each case you need to imagine lifting the decimal point off the paper and moving it.

Divide 250 by 1,000, pick up the decimal point and move it 3 places to drop it in front of the 2, e.g.

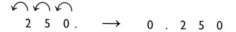

$$2\ 5\ 0\ .\quad \longrightarrow \quad 0\ .\ 2\ 5\ 0$$

Such conversions are required in medication dosage calculations; therefore you must be confident about them.

To change *larger units* (e.g. milligrams) to *smaller units* (e.g. micrograms) **multiply** the number by 1,000.

Or move the decimal point 3 places in this direction ⇦

To change *smaller units* (e.g. milligrams (mg)) to *larger units* (e.g. grams) **divide** the number by 1,000.

Or move the decimal point 3 places in this direction ⇨

For example:

1. To convert 5 grams (g) to milligrams (mg) **multiply by 1,000** = 5,000 mg (because (g) are bigger than (mg) and there are 1,000 milligrams in a gram).

2. To convert 6 litres (l) to millilitres (ml) **multiply by 1,000** = 6,000 ml (because (l) are bigger than (ml) and there are 1,000 millilitres in a litre).

3. To convert 16,000 micrograms (mcg) to milligrams (mg) **divide by 1,000** = 16 mg (because (mg) are bigger than micrograms (mcg) and there are 1,000 micrograms in a milligram).

Medication forms and calculations

Tablets or capsules act as a *vehicle* for the active constituents, which are measured in grams (g), milligrams (mg) or micrograms (mcg). By swallowing such tablets/capsules, the drugs can be absorbed into the bloodstream, to have an effect.

Some drugs are prepared in liquid forms and in this case the drug is dissolved in or suspended in a liquid such as water. Therefore the liquid is the *vehicle* for taking the drug into the body.

The drug will still be measured in grams (g), milligrams (mg) or micrograms (mcg) but because this drug is in liquid, it has a *concentration*: that is, a number of g, mg or mcg per ml of liquid, e.g. Furosemide 40 mg per 1 ml.

Use this formula for drug calculations

What you give = dose prescribed (what you want) ÷ dispensed dose (what you've got) x what it is in. Consider these examples:

Example 1

Dose prescribed is 150 mg/dispensed dose is 50 mg/which is in 5 ml.

Therefore the sum is 150 ÷ 50 x 5 = what you give = 15 ml

Example 2

Dose prescribed is 300 mg/dispensed dose is 150 mg/which is in 1 capsule.

Therefore the sum is 300 ÷ 150 x 1 = what you give = 2 capsules

In the case of medication calculations that involve tablets or capsules, of course *what it is in* will always be 1 (one), whereas with liquid medicines or injections it may not be.

A useful thing to know about is *cancelling down*. This helps with the sort of calculations shown.

The calculations could be laid out as

$$\frac{150}{50} \times 5 \quad \text{and} \quad \frac{300}{150} \times 1$$

The rule for cancelling down is that if you apply a multiplication or division to the top of an equation, such as these, **and** apply the *same* multiplication or division to the bottom of the equation, then you will not change the answer.

This can help simplify the sum. In Example 3, both the top of the equation and the bottom of the equation have been divided by 50. In Example 4, both the top of the equation and the bottom of the equation have been divided by 150.

Example 3 (divided by 50)

$$\frac{\overset{3}{\cancel{150}}}{\underset{1}{\cancel{50}}} \times 5 = 15$$

Example 4 (divided by 150)

$$\frac{\overset{2}{\cancel{300}}}{\underset{1}{\cancel{150}}} \times 1 = 2$$

You may find it useful to know how to divide using a process called *long division*.

This is illustrated with this medication dosage problem in Example 5.

Example 5

Dose prescribed is 90 mg/dispensed dose is 75 mg/which is in 5 ml.

Therefore the sum is 90 ÷ 75 x 5. This would be easy if we knew what 90 ÷ 75 equals, but it is not immediately clear what that is.

Step 1	Step 2	Step 3
75 goes into 90 once, with 15 left over	Now that whole numbers have been dealt with, put a decimal point and bring down a zero	Now the remainder of the sum is 150 ÷ 75, the answer is 1.2
$\begin{array}{r} 1 \\ 75\overline{)90} \\ -75 \\ \hline 15 \end{array}$	$\begin{array}{r} 1 \\ 75\overline{)90} \\ -75 \\ \hline 150 \end{array}$	$\begin{array}{r} 1.2 \\ 75\overline{)90} \\ -75 \\ \hline 150 \\ -150 \\ \hline 0 \end{array}$

Figure 10.1 Example of long division

A long division approach would be set out like Fig. 10.1. Consider this and you'll see that therefore the answer to $90 \div 75 \times 5 = 1.2 \times 5 = 6$ ml.

Incidently, this calculation could also have been approached by *cancelling down*. For this the steps are:

Example 6

Step 1: *what goes into 90 and into 75?* 5 does. $90 \div 5 = 18$; $75 \div 5 = 15$

Step 2: *what goes into 15 and into 5?* 5 does. $15 \div 5 = 3$; $5 \div 5 = 1$

Step 3: *what goes into 18 and into 3?* 3 does. $18 \div 3 = 6$; $3 \div 3 = 1$

$$\frac{\overset{\overset{6}{\cancel{18}}}{\cancel{90}}}{\underset{\underset{1}{\cancel{15}}}{\cancel{75}}} \times \frac{1}{\cancel{15}}$$

Practise your skills

Figure 10.2 provides ten practice calculations exercises using long division or cancelling down—practise these and before checking your answers consider that some will involve conversion from one SI unit to another. In each case, say what you would give if administering the 06:00 am dose. Try doing them without a calculator. Check your answers with a calculator and then consult the answers at the end of this chapter.

A few drugs (e.g. insulin and heparin) are measured in *units*. However, the approach is the same as in Fig. 10.2.

The calculations exercises in Fig. 10.3 require you to choose from three heparin strengths—what would you draw up and give? Try to undertake the calculation and then consult the answers at the end of this chapter.

Prescriptions for IV fluids

Any prescription for IV fluids will state an amount to be given over a number of hours.

Stage 1, the first step, is to work out how many millilitres (ml) per hour, by dividing the amount of fluid prescribed by the number of hours.

Example 7

Stage 1

1,000 ml over 12 hours $= 1,000 \div 12 = 83.33$ ml per hour

450 ml over 3 hours $= 450 \div 3 = 150$ ml per hour

1

REGULAR PRESCRIPTIONS			Time
Approved Name Digoxin	Start Date 04/07/11		06.00
Dose 0.125 mg	Route ORAL	Special Instructions	12.00
Signature & Date: H. Waterman 03/07/11			18.00

DIGOXIN
125 micrograms
in 1 tablet

2

REGULAR PRESCRIPTIONS			Time
Approved Name Dipyridamole	Start Date 04/07/11		06.00
Dose 150 mg	Route ORAL	Special Instructions	12.00
Signature & Date: H. Waterman 03/07/11			18.00

DIPYRIDAMOLE
25 milligrams
in 1 tablet

3

REGULAR PRESCRIPTIONS			Time
Approved Name Cefuroxine	Start Date 04/07/11		06.00
Dose 0.75 g	Route I.M.	Special Instructions	12.00
Signature & Date: H. Waterman 03/07/11			18.00

CEFUROXINE
750 milligrams
in 6 ml

4

REGULAR PRESCRIPTIONS			Time
Approved Name Ibuprofen	Start Date 04/07/11		06.00
Dose 120 mg	Route ORAL	Special Instructions	12.00
Signature & Date: H. Waterman 03/07/11			18.00

IBUPROFEN Syrup
100 milligrams
in 5 ml

5

REGULAR PRESCRIPTIONS			Time
Approved Name Ceftazidime	Start Date 04/07/11		06.00
Dose 1 g	Route I.V.	Special Instructions	12.00
Signature & Date: H. Waterman 03/07/11			18.00

CEFTAZIDIME
1 gram in 10 ml

6

REGULAR PRESCRIPTIONS			Time
Approved Name Nicotinic Acid	Start Date 04/07/11		06.00
Dose 200 mg	Route ORAL	Special Instructions	12.00
Signature & Date: H. Waterman 03/07/11			18.00

NICOTINIC ACID
50 milligrams
in 1 tablet

Figure 10.2 Practice calculations

7

REGULAR PRESCRIPTIONS			Time
Approved Name *Chlopromazine*		Start Date 04/07/11	06.00
Dose 75 mg	Route ORAL	Special Instructions	12.00
Signature & Date: H. Waterman 03/07/11			18.00

CHLOPROMAZINE
Syrup
25 milligrams
in 5 ml

8

REGULAR PRESCRIPTIONS			Time
Approved Name *Furosemide*		Start Date 04/07/11	06.00
Dose 40 mg	Route ORAL	Special Instructions	12.00
Signature & Date: H. Waterman 03/07/11			18.00

FUROSEMIDE
40 milligrams
in 1 tablet

9

REGULAR PRESCRIPTIONS			Time
Approved Name *Sulphasalazine*		Start Date 04/07/11	06.00
Dose 1 g	Route ORAL	Special Instructions	12.00
Signature & Date: H. Waterman 03/07/11			18.00

SULPHASALAZINE
Suspension
250 milligrams
in 5 ml

10

REGULAR PRESCRIPTIONS			Time
Approved Name *Paracetamol suspension*		Start Date 04/07/11	06.00
Dose 90 mg	Route ORAL	Special Instructions	12.00
Signature & Date: H. Waterman 03/07/11			18.00

PARACETAMOL
Suspension
120 milligrams
in 5 ml

Figure 10.2 (*continued*)

Prescription

Approved Name *Heparin*	
Dose 5000 units	Route s.c.

Available

HEPARIN 1,000 units per 1 ml	HEPARIN 5,000 units per 1 ml	HEPARIN 25,000 units per 1 ml

Figure 10.3 Calculations exercises

This is as far as you need to go, if you are using a volumetric pump. **Most acute settings use volumetric pumps and this is all the calculation needed.**

If, however, you need to calculate the rate for drops per minute, you need a second stage.

Stage 2 in the process is to divide the millilitres per hour by 60 to get the right number of millilitres per minute and to multiply by how many drops there are in each millilitre, as specified on the giving set packaging. This can be done as one *cancelling down* equation:

Example 8

Stage 2

$$\text{Formula: } \frac{\text{millilitres per hour} \times \text{drops per ml}}{60}$$

For example, when prescription says 1,000 ml over 8 hours and the giving set has 20 drops per ml

$$\frac{83.33 \times 20}{60}$$

The 20 and 60 can be used for cancelling down, leaving:

$$\frac{83.33}{3}$$

which is 28 drops per minute (to nearest whole drop).

If the infusion is to be administered in less than one hour, you need to adjust the method omitting the converting to minutes step and so not dividing by 60 (see Example 9).

Example 9

A patient is to receive 150 ml of saline (0.9%) over 40 minutes. The IV set delivers 20 drops/ml. At what rate (drops per minute) should the drip rate be set?

$$\text{Number of drops per minute} = \frac{150 \times 20}{40} \qquad (\text{or } 150 \times 20 \div 40)$$

that is, after cancelling down to $\frac{150}{2}$, the answer is 75 drops per minute.

As you can see, rounding up/down to a whole number of drops makes sense (round up 0.5 and above; round down 0.4 and below).

Practise your skills

Figure 10.4 has three IV infusion prescriptions. Consider the different calculations for each one and check your answers at the end of the chapter.

Question 1: Calculate
a) the number of millilitres per hour
b) the number of drops per minute, with the indicated giving set

Infusion Fluid			Infusion Duration
Type/Strength	Volume	Route	
Whole Blood	450 ml	I.V.	4 hours
Signature & Date: H. Waterman 03/07/11			

Giving set
Intravenous administration set
15 drops per ml

Question 2: Calculate
a) the number of millilitres per hour
b) the number of drops per minute, with the indicated giving set

Infusion Fluid			Infusion Duration
Type/Strength	Volume	Route	
Sodium Chloride 0.9%	1,000 ml	I.V.	8 hours
Signature & Date: H. Waterman 03/07/11			

Giving set
Intravenous administration set
12 drops per ml

Question 3: Calculate
a) the number of drops per minute, with the indicated giving set

Infusion Fluid			Infusion Duration
Type/ Strength	Volume	Route	
Sodium Chloride 0.9%	250 ml	I.V.	40 minutes
Signature & Date: H. Waterman 03/07/11			

Giving set
Intravenous administration set
60 drops per ml

Figure 10.4 Practice calculations

 # Online resource centre

You can find further advice and revision help for your OSCEs by going online now to see **www.oxfordtextbooks.co.uk/orc/caballero/.**

 # References

Hutton, B.M. et al. (2010). *Benchmark Assessment of Numeracy for Nursing: Medication Dosage Calculation at Point of Registration*. Edinburgh: NHS Education for Scotland.

Jukes, L. and Gilchrist, M. (2006). Concerns about numeracy skills of nursing students. *Nurse Education in Practice*, 6(4): 192–198.

National Patient Safety Agency (2009). *Safety in Doses: Improving the Use of Medicines in the NHS*. London: NPSA.

Nursing and Midwifery Council (2010). *Standards for Pre-Registration Nursing Education.* London: Nursing and Midwifery Council.

Sabin, M. (2001). *Competence in Practice-Based Calculation: Issues for Nursing Education. A Critical Review of the Literature.* Loughborough: The Learning and Teaching Support Network (LTSN).

 ## Appendix: answers to calculation exercises

Practise your skills (Fig. 10.2)

1. 1 tablet, *since 0.125 mg is equal to 125 mcg*
2. 6 tablets
3. 6 ml, *since 0.75 g is equal to 750 mg*
4. 1.2 ml
5. 10 ml
6. 4 tablets
7. 15 ml
8. 1 tablet
9. 20 ml
10. 3.75 ml

Practise your skills (Fig. 10.3)

5 ml of heparin 1,000 units per 1 ml

Or 1 ml of heparin 5,000 units per 1 ml

Or 0.2 ml of heparin 25,000 units per 1 ml (best option, since smallest injection)

Practise your skills (Fig. 10.4)

1. a: 112.5 ml/hour

   b: 28 drops/min
2. a: 125 ml/hour

   b: 25 drops/min
3. 375 drops/min

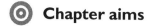

Chapter 11
Administration of oral medication
Fiona Creed

 Chapter aims

This chapter will enable you to:

- Understand why this important skill is assessed using OSCE,
- Revise key material in relation to this skill,
- Follow a step by step guide to the medication administration process,
- Understand how to prepare and revise for this OSCE,
- Highlight common problems at this station and identify how these may be avoided.

Introduction

Medication administration is a key skill and it is vital that you are able to demonstrate safety in all aspects of the medication administration process in order to avoid harm or death to your patient. The NMC (2004, 2010) reiterates this point, highlighting that the administration of medicines is an important aspect of a nurse's professional practice. They argue that it is not simply a mechanistic task, but one that requires thought, exercise and professional judgement.

Studies suggest that medicine administration is one of the highest risk processes that a nurse will undertake in clinical practice (NPSA 2007b; Elliot and Lui 2010). Medication administration errors are one of the most common errors reported to the National Patient Safety Agency (NPSA). Indeed in a 12-month period in 2007, 72,482 medication errors were reported with 100 of these causing either death or severe harm to the patient (NPSA 2009). The frequency of these errors has led to a number of changes in the medication administration process. Alongside these important recommendations, most higher education establishments will want to ensure safety of medicine administration and may test this vital skill using an OSCE to ensure that you are adequately prepared for safe administration of medication in practice.

Key revision for your simulated examination

General principles of medication administration

There are a number of important laws and key documents that relate to the administration of medication and it is important that you understand these as they all impact upon your practice when administering medication to a patient. You may also be tested on your knowledge in relation to these areas so it is important that you have read these. Important documents you will need to know include:

- The laws that relate to medication in the UK,
- NMC Standards for Medicines Management (2010) (www.nmc-uk.org),
- Local policies related to hospital/Primary Care Trust (PCT) regulation of medication (refer to local guidance).

Laws related to medication administration

There are a number of laws that influence the manufacturing, prescription, supply, storage and administration of medication. Whilst you will not need to study the intricacies of these laws you will need to understand the main issues each law covers. These are summarized in Table 11.1. You may be expected to answer questions in relation to one or more of these laws in your OSCE.

Professional regulations

The NMC provides extensive guidance that relates to medicines management. This document has increasingly expanded over the last decade as nurses take on a broader role in the prescription and administration of medication. The NMC provides guidance related to:

- Supply and administration of medication,
- Dispensing of medication,
- Storage and transport of medicines,
- Standards for the practice of administration of medication,
- Delegation of responsibility related to medication administration,
- Disposal of medicinal products,
- Use of unlicensed products,
- Use of complementary and alternative therapies,
- Errors in the administration of medication,
- Controlled drugs.

Note: Whilst this document is extremely large it is important that you understand this as it provides important guidance for both the student and registered practitioner. You may be expected to answer questions in relation to NMC guidance in your OSCE.

Local policies related to hospital/PCT regulation of medication

Alongside the laws and national and regulatory body guidance you will also have local policies that will guide your practice. It is important that you familiarize yourself with local policies as these can vary between NHS Trusts/PCTs and you will be expected to adhere to national and local guidance when administering medication.

Systematic medication administration

In order to avoid medication errors it is important that you follow a systematic method when administering medication as this will help to reduce the risk of medication error and promote patient safety (Shawyer and Endacott 2009). It is widely accepted that most medication errors are multifaceted

Table 11.1 **Laws related to medication**

Law	Key points that affect practice
Medicines Act (1968)	The first comprehensive legislation in the UK that provided a legal framework for the manufacturing, licensing, prescribing, supply and administration of medicines. The act classifies medication into: • Prescription only medicines, • Pharmacy only medicines, • General sales list medicines, • Controlled drugs.
Misuse of Drugs Act (1971)	Provides the statutory framework for control and regulation of controlled drugs. It defines a controlled drug as any drug listed in Schedule 2 of the Act.
Misuse of Drugs Regulations (1973)	Relates to storage of controlled drugs. The degree of control depends upon where medications are being stored. In hospitals this regulation stipulates that medicines must be in a locked cabinet or safe that is fixed to a wall.
Duthie Report (1988)	Requires all NHS Trusts to set up, document and maintain procedures to ensure medicine storage and handling is safe and secure. The report highlights the key role of ward manager in safe and secure medication storage.
Prescription Only Medicines Order (1997)	Sets out requirements for a valid prescription.
Misuse of Drugs Regulations (2001)	Classifies five schedules according to different levels of control required. Level 1 requires highest level of control whereas level 5 is much lower level of control. Medications in Schedule 1 have no recognized medicinal use. Most opiate based analgesia are listed under Schedule 2 of these regulations.
Health Act (2006)	Relates to health care organizations and highlighted that all organizations should appoint a designated accountable officer to regulate medication. This Act allows other bodies to share information. Allows power of entry by police to inspect stocks and records of controlled drugs.

and happen as a result of failures within the system that health care professionals work in (Cohen and Shastay 2008; NPSA 2007b). However, it is important to recognize that nurses are often the last person who can check for error prior to administration of medicine and have a vital role in the prevention of error.

> ✳ KEY POINT! Throughout this chapter the use of a systematic approach will be emphasized utilizing the '5 rights' approach to medication administration (Clayton 1987). This ensures that medication by whichever route it is administered is:

- Given to the right patient,
- The right drug,
- The right route,
- The right dose,
- Given at the right time.

Prevention of administration errors

Common errors have been linked to personal factors and systems errors and it is important that you have an awareness of this when administering medication.

A number of person centered factors have been identified (Jones 2009; Castledine 2009). These include:

- Poor numeracy skills by nurses (see Chapter 10),
- Poor adherence to protocol, in particular not stringently following the '5 rights' process,
- Not adequately checking patient (see section on right patient identification).

Equally a number of system factors have been identified that relate to the busyness of the ward situation, time pressures and frequent interruptions (Jones 2009). To this end a large number of NHS Trusts have implemented protected medication time to help reduce the number of errors.

Patient consent/education

As with all care in nursing, it is vital to gain patient consent prior to the administration of medication. More recently studies have suggested that it is important to provide information about the medication to the patient (Latter 2010). The purpose of this is twofold. Firstly it ensures that the patient is providing informed consent. Secondly understanding of the role and importance of medication increases patient compliance in self administering medication following discharge home from hospital (Latter 2010).

Infection control

Several steps must be considered throughout the administration of medicines that relate to infection control and it is important that the nurse follows correct infection control procedures.

Hands should be decontaminated using soap and water or alcohol rub (Dougherty and Lister 2008; Hatchett 2009). It is not normally necessary to wear gloves unless you are preparing intravenous medication, **intramuscular** injections or require gloves to protect yourself from body fluids, e.g nasogastric or rectal administration of medicines. Remember if your patient scenario involves administering medication to a patient with a transferable infection, e.g. MRSA, then **personal protective equipment** should be used in accordance with local policy.

Any medication administered should not be directly touched by the nurse (Hatchett 2009) and this will require you to practise a careful technique if the medication is stored in a bottle. You should also ensure that any equipment used for the administration of medication is free from sources of contamination, e.g. sterile syringes, sterile hypodermic needles and disposable medicine pots. Where advanced routes of medication are being used, e.g. intravenous administration, nurses should familiarize themselves with correct infection prevention technique.

Utilizing these approaches in your OSCE examination

In clinical practice there is a wide variety of methods used to administer medication to patients. It is important to find out which method you are being assessed on in your OSCE and you are advised to refer to your own university's OSCE coordinators for this information.

The purpose of this chapter is to enable you to systematically administer oral medication. If your OSCE relates to alternative routes of administration you can follow the same generic principles but will need to refer to an appropriate clinical skills book for revision of different methods of administration.

It is likely that you will be provided with a medication prescription chart and asked to administer medication to one patient as though you were a registered nurse (i.e. single nurse administration). It is most likely that you will be required to administer oral medication or perhaps a combination of oral medication/injections.

Whichever the approach you will be expected to:

- Provide sufficient information that your patient may give informed consent,
- Maintain infection control throughout,
- Systematically administer medication,
- Make any appropriate checks to the patient (e.g. check BP prior to administering anti-hypertensive medication),
- Document effectively,
- Discuss how you would monitor your patient post administration.

Remember you will be assessed on your:

- Professional attitude,
- Communication with the patient and other staff,
- Ability to administer medication systematically,
- Knowledge related to medication,
- Ability to maintain infection control,
- Documentation throughout the administration process.

Step by step

Systematic medication administration

Introduction and consent

It is vital that you introduce yourself to your patient and **explain** the need for the administration of medication. During this stage it is vital that you gain the patient's consent and provide information. You will also be required to provide more information in relation to the medication as you progress

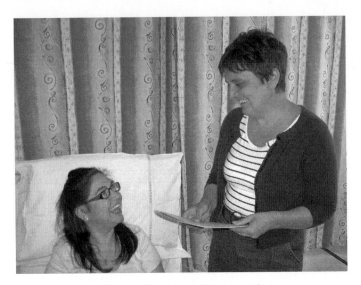

Figure 11.1a Introduce yourself

through the OSCE. It is essential to remember infection control and hands should be decontaminated (washed with soap and water or alcohol gel) prior to commencing medication administration. You will be expected to demonstrate a **professional attitude** to the patient throughout the administration process. Having clearly introduced yourself (see Fig. 11.1a) and maintained infection control you will then be required to systematically check and administer the medication.

Right patient

It is essential to ensure you are administering medication to the correct patient and recent directives reiterate the need to ensure that you have the correct patient (NPSA 2009; NMC 2010). **Remember** 10% of errors in medication are caused by neglecting to ensure the correct medication is given to the correct patient with 2,900 of these errors related to failure to check patient wristbands (NPSA 2007a, 2007b).

Current recommendation is to check the patient's identity using a patient wristband if the medication is being provided in an acute care setting (Fig. 11.1b). The NPSA (2007a) has called for standardization of information on patients' name bands and suggests that it should include patient name, date of birth and NHS number. If you are in mental health or a learning disability field of nursing you should ensure that you follow established guidelines related to checking the identity of the patient as it is unlikely that the patient/client will be wearing a patient identification bracelet. In some instances photographs may be used to help identify patients.

You are cautioned against asking 'Are you Mr Smith?' as this may be an unsafe method of confirming identity, especially in confused patients or where patients may have the same/similar surnames (Elliot and Lui 2010). You should also double check the patient's name on the drug chart.

Remember patients with allergies should have a red wristband that includes patient details in black ink; there is no requirement to put other information, e.g. the name of the allergy, on the band (NPSA 2007a). The presence of a red band should prompt you to take further action rather than highlight the medication the patient is allergic to (Fig. 11.1c).

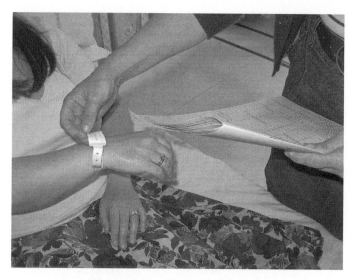

Figure 11.1b Check patient's identity

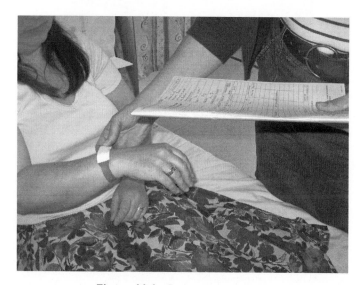

Figure 11.1c Red patient wristband

Right drug

It is estimated that 1/3 of medication errors are related to the wrong medication being administered (NPSA 2009). Therefore it is essential to ensure that you are administering the correct drug. You will need to ensure that the medication has been clearly and legibly prescribed by the prescriber (Fig. 11.1d). Recent evidence suggested that 14% of prescription charts had some form of error with several that could have potentially led to incorrect medication being administered (Simons 2010). **Remember** if the prescription is unclear in any way you should withhold the medication and speak to the prescriber and request that the prescription is rewritten in a legible manner (this will help

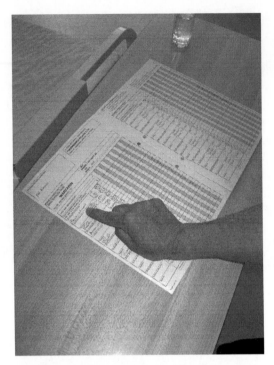

Figure 11.1d Check the prescription is legible

avoid further errors). When checking the chart you are also required to note any medication allergies and ensure that the patient is not allergic to any medication prescribed (NMC 2010). It is safe practice to always ask the patient about any allergies in addition to checking the medication chart.

In addition to checking the legibility and potential risk of allergy you will also need to **know** what the medication action is. It is vital to know this as it may be necessary to complete appropriate checks or review results prior to the medication being administered. For example you may be required to check blood pressure prior to administration of an antihypertensive medicine or need to check the patient's current potassium levels prior to the administration of oral potassium supplements. **Remember** you are not required to rote learn medications but you must demonstrate safe practice by checking the medication in action and required checks in a medication formulary, e.g. the BNF (Fig. 11.1e).

Remember there may well be deliberate medication prescribing errors on the chart in your OSCE to test your ability to act upon an incorrect prescription.

Alongside **knowledge** of medication action you may also be expected to demonstrate understanding of its benefits, contraindications and **side effects** of the medication you are administering (Hatchett 2009). You may be required to explain these either to your patient or to the examiner. This information can again be found in a medication formulary and you will not be expected to rote learn it. It is likely that the medication formulary will be available to you throughout your OSCE.

Communication will be a vital part of this aspect of administration and you will also be expected to explain the action of the medication and the benefits and potential side effects of taking the medication to your patient (Fig. 11.1f). Studies suggest that a patient's compliance with medication at discharge is affected by their understanding of the need for the medication so the nurse is expected to demonstrate appropriate patient education throughout the procedure and **communicate** this effectively with the patient (Latter 2010).

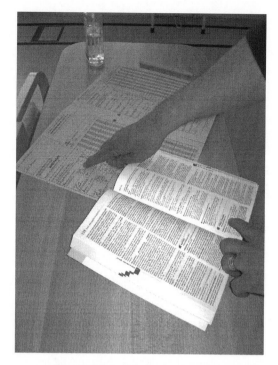

Figure 11.1e Medication formulary

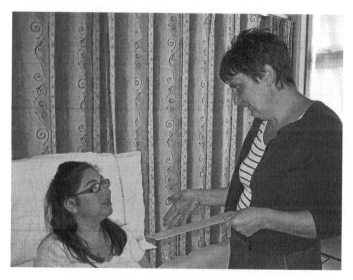

Figure 11.1f Communication

Right route

Nurses are increasingly required to administer medication via several routes and it is important that you are aware of and utilize the correct route for the medication. You should also be aware that changes in route may alter the dosage of the medication (e.g. morphine if given intravenously is given in a much smaller dose than if given intramuscularly). There have also been examples where medication intended for oral use has been administered via the intravenous route causing harm to the patient (Cohen 2006). **Remember** if you are administering any oral medication that requires very accurate measurement in a syringe you must utilize a blue oral medication syringe to help prevent any errors in inadvertent IV administration.

If your OSCE involves giving medication via different routes it is important to ensure that you understand how to administer the medication via that route and any necessary interventions that are required (e.g. left side lying for administration of rectal suppositories (Dougherty and Lister 2008)). You should discuss with your tutors which routes are likely to be utilized in your examination and revise these using an appropriate skills book.

Right time

Medication will be prescribed to be given at a set time and it is essential in your OSCE that you demonstrate your understanding of this important principle. The guiding principle is that medication should be administered as close to the prescribed time as possible (Elliot and Lui 2010). In clinical practice timing errors often relate to the incorrect timing of antibiotic therapy (Tang et al. 2007). Many medication actions are affected by the time span between doses and in medication such as antibiotics it is vital that they are given at specific times to ensure efficacy of serum antibiotic concentration.

It is suggested that medication is administered within half an hour of the prescribed time and if this is not possible, for whatever reason, a medication error should be reported and appropriate electronic or paper forms completed. You will also be expected to demonstrate other factors relating to timing of the medication, e.g. some medications such as steroids should ideally be taken with food to prevent potential stomach ulceration whilst some antibiotics need to be administered before food to facilitate absorption. Failure to demonstrate understanding of this in your OSCE will either prevent a pass grade being awarded or substantially reduce the mark you are awarded.

You will also need to demonstrate your ability to **explain** this to the patient in your OSCE as patients need to understand the need to take their medication at regular intervals, rather than at convenient times. Again the nurse is expected to demonstrate appropriate patient education throughout the procedure and **communicate** this effectively with the patient (Latter 2010).

Right dose

Administration of the correct dose of the medication is vital. However, studies suggest that the majority of medication errors relate to incorrect dosage (NPSA 2007b; Jones 2009). Whilst it is still generally medics who prescribe medication to acute patients (Jones 2009), nurses still have a professional responsibility to ensure that the dose prescribed is correct and should check this carefully with a medication formulary if they are unsure, before administering any medication (NMC 2010).

Nurses also have a responsibility to ensure that correct medication calculations are performed accurately. Problems associated with the nurse's ability to perform accurate medication calculation are well documented (Wright 2006; NPSA 2007; Lee 2008). The need for accurate medication calculations and improvement in nurse's confidence with arithmetic is emphasized throughout the literature (Wright 2006; Jones 2009). You are referred to Chapter 10 for additional detail on medication calculations.

The NMC (2010) also highlights the need for complex calculations to be checked by two trained nurses as the likelihood of error increases with the complexity of calculation. It highlights that although nurses may use calculators for complex medication calculations they should not replace accurate arithmetic knowledge and skill (NMC 2010).

Documentation

You will be expected to provide clear documentation in relation to medication administration and it is important that it is clearly documented which medications have been administered. It is also vital to correctly identify where medications have been withheld. The NMC highlights the need to provide **clear, accurate** and **immediate** record of all medication administered, intentionally withheld or refused by the patient. The documentation should be legible and clearly identify the person/persons responsible for the administration of medication.

You are advised to document that medication has been taken immediately after the patient takes the medication. Documentation prior to administration may cause problems if the patient refuses the medication. More worryingly failure to document that medication has been administered may result in the patient receiving the medication twice and result in potential harm to the patient (Elliot and Lui 2010). **Remember** you are required to witness that the patient actually takes the medication and medication should not be left with the patient to be taken later (Fig. 11.1g). Once taken, complete the drug chart (Fig. 11.1h).

Where medication is withheld or refused it is vital that the rationale for the decision to withhold or refusal is clearly documented on the patient's medication chart. For example where digoxin is withheld in a bradycardic patient the rationale related to low pulse should be clearly documented. It may also be necessary to refer the patient to the medical team if digoxin levels need to be taken, and again this should be clearly documented in the patient's medical/nursing record.

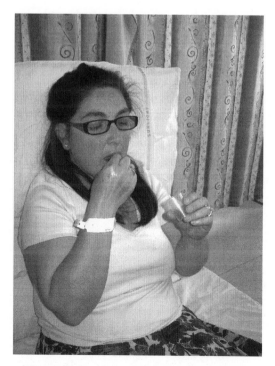

Figure 11.1g Witness patient taking medication

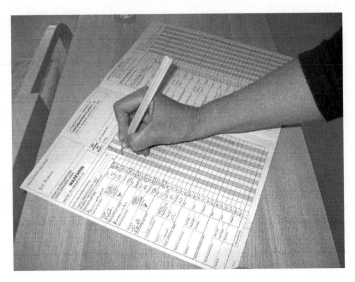

Figure 11.1h Complete drug chart

Any observations related to the administration of medication should also be clearly documented on the patient's observation chart so that it is apparent that appropriate checks have been made prior to the administration of medicines.

Some medications may require you to complete additional paperwork, e.g. if you are required to administer controlled medication you will be required to complete the necessary controlled medication documentation (Misuse of Drugs Regulations 1973, 2001).

Aftercare of patient

Once medication has been administered the nurse has a continuing **professional responsibility** to ensure that the patient receives appropriate aftercare (Elliot and Lui 2010). The nurse will need to perform any necessary checks following administration of medication (examples of these are included in Table 11.2).

Alongside appropriate observations the nurse should also observe the patient for any potential side effects or allergic reaction. You may be asked to explain how you would monitor for side effects and allergic reaction. It is useful to familiarize yourself with management of these situations and you are referred to the Resuscitation Council's (2008) guidance on the management of **anaphylaxis,** which you should know if you are involved in administering any form of medication. **Remember** patients may react to a new medication or one that they have taken before!

Safe storage of the medication

Following correct administration of medication you will be expected to ensure that medication is stored appropriately and in accordance with the manufacturer's recommendations (NMC 2010). The type of storage will vary and may reflect storage at the local NHS Trust, e.g. patient pod systems or more rarely medication trolleys. You will be expected to be able to state how medication should be correctly stored and may be expected to discuss laws that relate to the safe storage of medicines.

Table 11.2 **Aftercare following the administration of medication**

Medication	Aftercare required
Opiate based analgesia e.g. morphine	Regular physiological observation monitoring with emphasis on respiratory assessment. Appropriate pain assessment to ensure efficacy of medication.
Insulin	Blood glucose levels should be recorded before and after administration of subcutaneous insulin in hospitalized patients. Patients should be observed for signs and symptoms of hypoglycaemia and hyperglycaemia.
Salbutamol	Peak flow measurement should be recorded prior to administration and after administration to determine efficacy of medication in patients with acute exacerbation of their asthma. Accurate respiratory assessment should be performed to note for worsening or improving respiratory function.

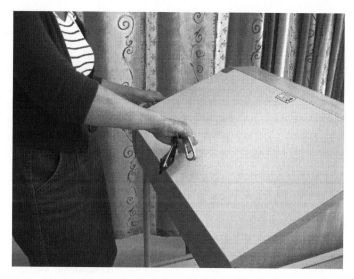

Figure 11.1i Safe storage of medication

With the exception of a few medications (e.g. cardiac arrest drugs and intravenous fluids) most drugs should be locked securely in a cupboard when not in use (Duthie Report 1988). You should therefore ensure that any medication used in the OSCE is returned to a secure cupboard (Fig. 11.1i).

Putting it all together!

An overview of systematic medication administration can be seen in Box 11.1 which provides a useful recap of all aspects of this skill.

Box 11.1 **Putting it all together!**

- Introduce yourself to the patient.
- Gain consent where able.
- Wash/gel your hands.
- Ensure you have all the equipment needed and the correct medication chart is available.
- Check the patient's name band to ensure patient and medication chart are correct.
- Check for signs of allergy by asking patient and reviewing medication chart/name band.
- Read through the chart initially to see if any medication is due and review to see if any tests, e.g. blood glucose, are required prior to administration of the medication.
- Check that you have the **right** drug that is prescribed on the chart. **Remember** the examiner will expect you to be able to describe the actions of the medication.
- Check that you are giving the medication by the correct route.
- Check that you are giving the medication at the correct time.
- Calculate the dose and double check this to ensure you are confident that the dose is correct.
- Ensure that a full explanation is given to the patient and that they understand why they are receiving the medication and explain the action of the drug in terms the patient will understand.
- Once you are confident that you have completed all the required checks, administer the medication.
- When you have observed that the patient has taken the medication accurately document this on the medication chart.
- Check that the patient is comfortable and check whether the patient requires any aftercare following administration of the medication and record this as required.
- Ensure the medication is returned to safe storage.

 Examiners' marking criteria

Various tools will be utilized to assess your competence at administration of medication. As stated in earlier chapters it is advisable to review your own university's marking criteria. An example of marking criteria is included in Table 11.3.

Table 11.3 **Example of examiners' marking criteria**

Student's name and cohort year	
Expected performance criteria	Demonstrated Yes/No
Student introduces themselves to the patient.	
Student decontaminates hands with alcohol gel or washes hands. Student uses appropriate personal protective equipment if this is required.	
Student explains the need to check medication chart and administer medication.	

Table 11.3 (continued)

Student's name and cohort year	
Expected performance criteria	Demonstrated Yes/No
Student gains consent to administer medication from the patient.	
Right patient checks: • Student checks patient's name on wristband against the name, date of birth and NHS hospital number on the medication chart. • Student checks to see if patient is wearing an allergy band and also if any allergies are noted on medication chart.	
Right drug checks: • Student checks that prescription is legible and that instructions are clear and follow NHS and local protocols. • Student identifies the medication that is due at that time. • Student rechecks that any medication that is due does not provide an allergy for the patient. • Student demonstrates understanding of medications by discussing the following: **indication** for medication, possible contraindications and side effects. • Student explains the use of the medication to the patient and checks their understanding. • The student explains to the patient any checks that may be required before the medication is administered, e.g. taking pulse prior to administration of digoxin. • The student performs any tests that are necessary and documents them clearly on appropriate paperwork, e.g. blood pressure on observation chart.	
Right route checks: • The student explains the route that the medication is to be given by to the examiner. • The student checks that the dose is correct for the selected route. • If medication is not oral the student should explain to the examiner how the medication will be administered and any necessary precautions in this route: e.g. how to avoid the sciatic nerve when administering intramuscular injections. • The student explains the route selected to the patient when the medication is ready for administration.	
Right time checks: • Student checks the time that the medication is due. • Student checks any issues that may relate to timing, e.g. administering medication before food or with food/glass of milk. • Student explains the need to take medication regularly as prescribed to the patient in order to maintain effective therapeutic blood levels of that medication where this is required, e.g. antibiotic therapy. • Student checks expiry date on medication.	

(continued)

Table 11.3 *(continued)*

Student's name and cohort year	
Expected performance criteria	Demonstrated Yes/No

Right dose checks:
  • Student calculates medication dose accurately.
  • Student explains calculation to examiner.
  • Student places appropriate dose of medication in pot using a non-touch technique, prior to administration to the patient.	

Administration of medicines:
  • The student checks all medications to be dispensed using the 5 rights method.
  • Once all medications are dispensed in pot the student gives the medication to the patient, again explaining rationale for medication and rechecking consent.
  • The student observes the patient taking the medication.	

Documentation:
  • The student documents that medication has been administered on the medication chart immediately, ensuring that signatures are clear and accurate and follow local and NHS guidance.
  • The student documents clearly and accurately any medications that have been withheld/not administered or refused by the patient and follows local policy to complete appropriate paperwork.	

Patient aftercare:
  • The student performs any observations/test that are required following administration of medication; for example post administration blood pressure following administration of ACE inhibitors.
  • The student observes the patient for signs of side effects and potential allergic reactions.	

Safe storage • Student secures medication safely following administration of medication.	
Please indicate Refer/Pass for skill	
Please indicate Refer/Pass for knowledge	

🗨 Examiners' questions

Some universities may assess your knowledge in relation to administration of medication and it is useful to prepare for that if that is a requirement. Box 11.2 outlines some typical questions.

> ### Box 11.2 **Example of examiners' questions**
>
> 1. Identify two reasons why it is important to administer drugs and not leave on patient's bedside.
> 2. Identify two different types of practitioners who can prescribe medication.
> 3. Identify two controlled drugs and state why these drugs are controlled.
> 4. Identify three symptoms of anaphylaxis.
> 5. Explain the limitation of the student nurse's role in the administration of medication.
> 6. Identify three actions to take if patient suffers anaphylactic reaction.
> 7. Describe how controlled drugs should be stored in a hospital environment.
> 8. Describe how you would gain consent for medication.
> 9. Discuss how you would document a medication that has been withheld.
> 10. Discuss how you would monitor for reactions.

Answers are provided at the end of the chapter.

✗ Common errors at this station

This may be a stressful station to undertake as students often have concerns over medication administration and a number of errors occur; these include problems related to failure to:

- Introduce yourself and communicate with the patient,
- Maintain infection control measures,
- Gain consent from the patient,
- Appropriately check the patient,
- Follow NPSA guidance to check patient's identify,
- Check for any allergies,
- Demonstrate sufficient knowledge of medication,
- Check in a medication formulary if at all unsure,
- Deliver correct medication dosage,
- Utilize correct medication calculation,
- Observe patient taking medication,
- Record appropriate observations before administration of medicine,
- Record appropriate observations after administration of medicine,
- Document appropriately.

Alongside these, other common errors include:

- Making assumptions that the medication chart will correctly prescribe doses, times and routes of medicines. Remember there may be deliberate errors,
- Panicking and becoming stressed,
- Rushing administration and making errors.
- Poor communication with the patient,
- Poor timing in the station/running out of time.

Top tips for passing this station

The key to passing this exam station is demonstrating the ability to:

- Follow a systematic approach when administering medication.
- Take time to ensure you have read and understood the medication chart and associated medications.
- Use the BNF to check medications; you are not expected to know the mechanisms of actions of all the medication you are asked to administer but MUST demonstrate safety in checking when unsure.
- Remember to check the patient's name band.
- Double check any calculations you may be required to perform.
- Communicate with your patient throughout, offering explanations at an appropriate level.
- Perform any necessary safety checks/after checks as these will demonstrate your understanding of the need for safety and mechanism of the drug action.

You may enhance your ability to pass this station by practising this skill and there are several things that students have found helpful:

- Practising alongside your colleagues in clinical skills room,
- Attending university practice and theory sessions,
- Using the skill in practice with your mentor and asking for constructive feedback,
- Attending study sessions that are run in practice (if the NHS Trust allows this),
- Practising sequence whilst being timed; this allows you to roughly calculate how much time is needed for each part of the assessment,
- Checking with your university lecturers which routes of administration will be used in the OSCE.

 ## Online resource centre

You can find further advice and revision help for your OSCEs by going online now to see www.oxfordtextbooks.co.uk/orc/caballero/.

References

Castledine, G. (2009) Blasé about drug administration. *British Journal of Nursing,* 18(19): 1219.

Clayton, M. (1987). The right way to prevent medicines errors. *Registered Nurse,* (50): 30–31.

Cohen, H. and Shastay, A. (2008). Getting to the root of medication errors. *Nursing,* 38(12): 39–47.

Cohen, M. (2006). Medication error: unfamiliar syringe, wrong route. *Nursing,* 36(3): 39–47.

Dougherty, L. and Lister, S. (2008). *The Royal Marsden Hospital Manual of Clinical Nursing Procedures, Student Edn.* Chichester: Wiley Blackwell.

Duthie Report (1988). The Safe and Secure Handling of Medicine: A Team Approach. London: Royal Pharmaceutical Society.

Elliot, M. and Lui, Y. (2010). The nine rights of drug administration: an overview. *British Journal of Nursing,* 19(5): 300–305.

Hatchett, R. (2009). Administration of medication. Clinical skills.net.

Jones, S. W. (2009). Reducing medication administration errors in nursing practice. *Nursing Standard*, 23(50): 40–46.

Latter, S. (2010). Evidence base for effective medicines management. *Nursing Standard* 24(43): 62–66.

National Patient Safety Agency (2007a). *Standardizing Wristbands Improves Patient Safety.* London: NPSA.

National Patient Safety Agency (2007b). *Safety in Doses: Medication Safety Incidents in the NHS: The Fourth Report from the Patient Safety Agency.* London: NPSA.

National Patient Safety Agency (2009). *Safety in Doses: Improving the Use of Medicines in the NHS.* London: NPSA.

Nursing and Midwifery Council (2004). *Guidelines for the Administration of Medicines.* London: NMC.

Nursing and Midwifery Council (2010). *Standards for Medicines Management.* London: NMC.

Resuscitation Council (UK) (2008). *Emergency Treatment of Anaphylactic Reactions: Guidelines for Healthcare Providers.* London: Resuscitation Council.

Shawyer, V. and Endacott, R. (2009). Drug administration. In: Endacott, R., Jevon, P. and Cooper, S. (2009) *Clinical Nursing Skills, Core and Advanced.* Oxford: Oxford University Press.

Simons, J. (2010). Identifying medication errors in surgical prescription charts. *Paediatric Nursing,* 22(5): 20–23.

Tang, F., Sheu, S., Wei, I. and Chen, C. (2007). Nurses relate the contributing factors involved in medication errors. *Journal of Clinical Nursing,* 16(3): 447–557.

Wright, K. (2006). Barriers to accurate drug calculations. *Nursing Standard,* 20(28): 41–45.

Appendix: answers to examiners' questions

1. Identify two reasons why it is important to administer drugs and not leave on patient's bedside
   - Patient may forget to take medication,
   - Medication should be taken at prescribed time,
   - Patient may knock drugs on floor,
   - Risk to other patients, especially the confused patients,
   - You are signing to say you have witnessed the patient swallow medication,
   - Patient may store drugs,
   - Risk of attempted suicide in depressed patients.

2. Identify practitioners who can prescribe drugs
   - Doctors,
   - Dentists,
   - Nurses (limited),
   - Pharmacists (limited),
   - Midwives (limited).

3. Identify two controlled drugs and state why these are controlled
   for controlled drugs see BNF
   Reasons include:
   - Dangerous,
   - Harmful,
   - Potentially addictive or habit forming.

4. Identify three symptoms of anaphylaxis
   - Extreme anxiety,
   - Feeling of impending doom,
   - Skin itching/flushing/urticaria,
   - Tachycardia,
   - Hypotension,
   - Airway obstruction,
   - Swelling,
   - Wheezing/stridor/dyspnoea,
   - Eventual cardiac and **respiratory arrest.**

5. Explain limitation of the student nurse's role in administration of medication
   - Can only dispense drugs in presence of registered nurse,
   - Cannot be involved in single nurse drug administration,
   - Must have drug administration countersigned by a registered practitioner,
   - Must also follow NHS Trust guidelines.

6. Identify three actions to take if patient suffers anaphylactic reaction
   - Seek urgent medical help,
   - Prepare drugs: adrenalin, chlorpheniramine, hydrocortisone,
   - Maintain airway,
   - Administer oxygen,
   - Check vital signs,
   - Reassure patient,
   - Prepare to use resuscitation equipment if needed.

7. Controlled drugs should be stored:
   - Double locked cupboard,
   - Separate key,
   - Ward sister or deputy should hold keys,
   - Ward sister or deputy accountable for keys.

8. Consent
   - Verbal consent should be gained from the patient,
   - Where this is not possible in the case of an unconscious patient or where there are mental capacity issues students should follow guidance from the Mental Capacity Act,
   - Under no circumstances should students administer medication covertly.

9. Withheld drugs
   Local policy should be followed, such as:
   - Writing rationale in appropriate area on medication chart,
   - Using code on medication chart to identify rationale,
   - The nurse in charge and doctor responsible for the patient should be informed.

10. Reactions
    - Observation of the patient required,
    - Patient may require recording of physiological observations,
    - The nurse should be conversant with potential side effects of particular medication and discuss how these will be monitored,
    - The nurse should be conversant with signs of allergic reaction and monitor for these.

Chapter 12
Recognition of acute deterioration
Fiona Creed

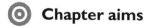

 Chapter aims

This chapter will enable you to:

- Understand why this advanced skill is assessed using OSCE,
- Revise key material in relation to this skill,
- Follow a step by step guide to the patient assessment process,
- Understand how to prepare and revise for this OSCE,
- Highlight common problems at this station and identify how these may be avoided.

Introduction

Recognition and prompt treatment of the acutely ill patient is a significant issue in clinical practice (NICE 2007). The need for all nurses to be able to recognize, assess and promptly escalate (ensure timely and effective management) patients whose condition is deteriorating is stressed in the literature (NCEPOD 2005; NPSA 2007). Therefore it is an important skill and your university will want to ensure via OSCE that you are adequately prepared for any emergency that may arise in practice.

It must be emphasized that this skill is a **complex skill** and most universities do not assess this skill until the **final year** of your course. The key to succeeding in this OSCE is understanding the need for systematic assessment, and timely intervention and **escalation** will be stressed throughout this chapter. It is likely that you will be allowed approximately half an hour to demonstrate this skill and answer related questions.

Revision of key material will enable you to understand why assessment is important and provide you with a systematic framework to use in the OSCE and in clinical practice.

Key revision for your simulated examination

Problems with assessment

Concern over NHS staff's management of the deteriorating patient has been highlighted in the literature since the late 1990s. McQuillan *et al.* (1998) first discussed the concept of **suboptimal care** suggesting that often deterioration in patients was ignored, misdiagnosed and/or poorly managed in ward environments resulting in increased mortality and morbidity in ward patients.

Since McQuillan's work several other studies have identified similar problems (McGloin *et al.* 1999; NCEPOD 2005). More recently NICE (2007) has published guidance on recognition and management of deterioration and the Department of Health (2009) has published competencies related to recognition and management of deterioration that all acute staff should achieve.

Review of this literature highlights that several issues are clearly important in recognition of acute deterioration and the need to utilize a systematic assessment tool linked to a robust **track and trigger scoring system** is an important consideration in practice.

ALERT ®: a systematic assessment tool

Smith (2003) was instrumental in developing the ALERT® framework that has been adopted internationally as a robust systematic assessment tool. The framework encourages practitioners to utilize a systematic approach to assessment based on an alphabetical approach that is adapted from the resuscitation framework (Creed *et al.* 2010).

This systematic tool focuses upon assessment of:

- Airway,
- Breathing,
- Circulation,
- Disability,
- Exposure/Everything else/Escalation.

The tool encourages practitioners to use a stepwise (systematic and logical framework) tool that focuses upon recognition of potentially life threatening problems first using a 'look, listen and feel' approach (Jevon 2007). Practitioners are encouraged to recognize and treat any problem before continuing with the assessment, e.g. if a problem is noted in breathing this should be addressed before assessment of circulation continues. One example of this could be the addition of oxygen in a patient with increasing respiratory rate and decreasing saturations. The application of oxygen would be instigated before the practitioner continued with cardiovascular assessment.

Track and trigger scoring systems

Alongside the need for immediate systematic patient assessment most assessments will require you to calculate a track and trigger score that facilitates identification of acute deterioration and promotes rapid patient escalation. Most NHS Trusts have followed the NICE (2007) guidelines and implemented track and trigger scoring systems. Many differing scoring systems are used but all focus on attributing a score that increases as the patient's condition worsens and their observations fall outside of normal ranges. Track and trigger systems may be referred to locally as patient at risk scores (PARS), early warning scores (EWS) or modified early warning scores (MEWS).

In 2007 NICE identified key components of all track and trigger scoring systems and emphasized the need to include the following parameters:

- Heart rate,
- Respiratory rate,
- Systolic blood pressure,
- Level of consciousness,
- Oxygen saturations,
- Temperature.

See Box 12.1 for a reminder of normal parameters and examples of how to use a track and trigger system.

> ## Box 12.1 Reminders and examples of how to use a track and trigger system

1. Reminders of normal parameters

Normal parameters are generally accepted as:

- Heart rate 60–100 bpm,
- Respiratory rate 12–20 bpm,
- Systolic blood pressure 100–139 mmHg,
- Diastolic blood pressure 60–90 mmHg,
- Temperature 35.5–37.5,
- Oxygen saturations 94–98%.

Endacott et al. (2009);
British Thoracic Society (2008)

2. How to use a track and trigger scoring system

Track and trigger scoring systems will score 0 if parameters are normal but will record a point value if there is variation from the normal

▶ Example 1—John Smith
Heart rate 78
Respiratory rate 14
Systolic blood pressure 110
Temperature 37.1
Oxygen saturations 94:

Would most likely score 0

▶ Example 2—Jennifer Smith
Heart rate 103
Respiratory rate 20
Systolic blood pressure 110
Temperature 37.5
Oxygen saturations 94:

Would most likely score 2

Some scoring systems also utilize other parameters including:

- Pain assessment,
- Fluid balance,
- Urine output,
- Blood glucose level.

Escalation of concern

All track and trigger systems should be linked to an appropriate escalation policy that will facilitate timely and effective management of the patient whose condition is deteriorating. The escalation policy may prompt you to:

- Increase the frequency of observations,
- Call a medical practitioner (F1/F2/ SPR),
- Call for an emergency response. Such examples include critical care outreach teams (CCO), patient at risk teams (PART) and medical emergency team (MET).

Effective communication

The need to communicate effectively when escalating the patient is also important. Several tools have been developed to improve communication between nurses and doctors as studies have suggested that poor communication may prevent timely intervention and treatment (NCEPOD 2005; NPSA 2007). One example of an effective communication strategy is the SBAR tool developed by the NHS Institute for Innovation and Improvement (2008). This tool encourages nurses to state:

- Situation
    - Identify yourself and ward area,
    - State patient's name and rationale for calling,
    - State concern.
- Background
    - Provide patient history,
    - Identify reason for admission,
    - Give a brief overview of treatment to date.
- Assessment
    - Provide assessment utilizing a systematic approach (ABCDE),
    - Identify track and trigger score,
    - Suggest any suspicions you may have about the patient.
- Recommendation
    - Explain what you would like the doctor to do,
    - Give a time frame for patient review,
    - Document who you have spoken to and their response.

Utilizing these approaches in your OSCE examination

Overview

It is likely that you will be asked to assess and effectively manage a deteriorating patient using a simulation manikin in a pre-programmed scenario. Some universities may use 'actors' instead of manikins. You are advised to check your university guidelines as some may assess this skill formatively using groups of students whilst others may assess individual students using either a summative or formative approach. Whichever the approach the commonalties are:

- You will receive a patient handover and then be expected to assess your patient,
- You will be required to use a systematic tool and initiate first line management,
- You will be required to calculate a track and trigger score,
- You will demonstrate an ability to follow escalation protocols,
- You will communicate effectively with the patient throughout,
- You will demonstrate an ability to communicate your concerns about the patient,
- You will document effectively throughout the scenario.

Remember you will be assessed on your:

- Professional attitude,
- Communication with the patient and other staff,
- Ability to assess the patient systematically,
- Knowledge related to assessment,
- Ability to maintain infection control,
- Documentation throughout the assessment.

Step by step systematic assessment

Once introduced to the patient, you will be expected to follow a systematic framework and should demonstrate your ability to assess and initially manage the patient using a stepwise approach. It is important that you remember **infection control,** even in a potential emergency. You should decontaminate your hands prior to patient contact by either using alcohol hand gel or washing your hands with soap and water.

Airway

If your patient is able to talk to you this normally indicates a clear airway; however, you should not take this for granted and state that you will assess the airway. The patient's airway should be assessed for any signs of obstruction using a look, listen and feel approach (Fig. 12.1a). You will need to observe for complete or partial obstruction of the airway. If the airway is completely obstructed you will see no chest movement in the patient, no noise will be apparent (silent) and you will not be able to feel movement of air. If the airway is partially obstructed you may notice distressed breathing, e.g. paradoxical chest movement (see-saw breathing) and the workload of breathing will be significantly increased. You should be able to feel some degree of air entry/exit and there will be associated abnormal respiratory sounds, e.g. snoring, stridor, gurgling or wheezing.

If there are any problems associated with the airway these should be rectified appropriately before breathing is assessed. This may necessitate changing the patient's position or use of an artificial airway adjunct, e.g. insertion of a Guedel airway or nasopharyngeal airway (Jevon 2007). Selection of airway adjunct may be dependent upon the patient's consciousness levels as some patients may not tolerate a Guedel airway and a nasopharyngeal airway may be more appropriate, providing there is no history of skull fracture (Creed *et al.* 2010).

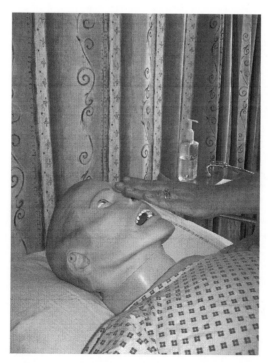

Figure 12.1a Assess for signs of obstruction using the look, listen and feel approach

Breathing

The patient's breathing should be assessed using a look, listen and feel approach (see Fig. 12.1b). The depth and inclusion of aspects of respiratory assessment may vary locally and care should be taken to familiarize yourself with what is required.

All assessments will require you to count the patient's respiratory rate for a whole minute (so ensure that you do count the respirations for a whole minute!). During this time you should observe:

- Pattern of respiration,
- Use of accessory muscles,
- Depth of respiration,
- Workload of breathing,
- Symmetry of breathing,
- Bilateral chest movement.

Some of these elements, e.g. use of accessory muscles, cannot be assessed in a manikin but you may be expected to ask the examiner about the presence of these. If any abnormalities are noted you should assess for dyspnoea by asking the patient if their breathing feels difficult. You should also note any obvious breathing noises, e.g. wheezing, stridor or persistent coughing.

Check   You should observe for signs of central cyanosis, bluish tinge to lips and mucous membranes around the mouth, again this cannot be assessed in a manikin but you may be expected to ask the examiner about the presence of cyanosis. You should ask the examiner about the colour of the patient's lips/mucous membranes.

Some universities may require you to perform more in-depth respiratory assessment which may include chest auscultation (listening to the lung fields using a stethoscope) (see Fig. 12.1c) and palpation (feeling for abnormalities such as tactile fremitus or the ability to feel secretions when the patient

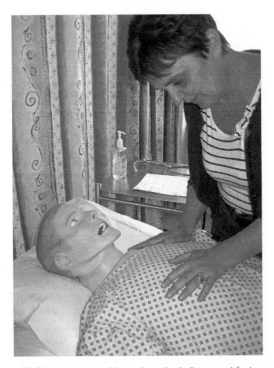

Figure 12.1b Assess breathing using a look, listen and feel approach

breathes). Others may also include percussion of the chest (tapping the chest wall to note resonance of air in the lung fields).

! *Note!*: Adequate respiratory assessment is a vital aspect of patient assessment as this will be the first observation to show signs of change during episodes of acute deterioration. The respiratory system will provide an early physiological warning that the patient's condition is deteriorating as the rate will quickly increase if there are respiratory or metabolic disturbances.

✱ KEY POINT! Studies have highlighted that changes in respiration are the most sensitive indicator of deterioration (Cretikos *et al*. 2008). Worryingly they are the most frequently omitted observation (NPSA 2007; Cretikos *et al*. 2008).

If the respiratory assessment identifies any difficulties the following measures may be considered:

- Emergency call if no or minimal respiratory effort,
- Change in patient's position to facilitate breathing,
- Application of oxygen following the British Thoracic Society guidance (2008),
- Reassurance for the patient,
- Encouragement of deep breathing,
- Use of medication, e.g. nebulization of bronchodilators if there is an expiratory wheeze on auscultation,
- Encouraging patient to cough if sputum retention evident on auscultation,
- Review of medication to see if patient has had any opiate based analgesia that may suppress respiration (or recreational drugs if A&E patient).

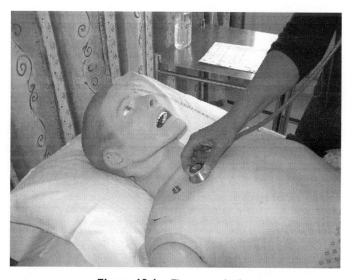

Figure 12.1c Chest auscultation

RR	12	14	15
O₂ Sats	98	94	90
O₂	A	2L	4L

Figure 12.2 Numerical recording

Document   You will also be required to record oxygen saturations and document respiratory rate and saturations on your patient observation chart. Some charts will require you to provide a numerical figure (see Fig. 12.2) whereas others may require a dot to be plotted in an appropriate area.

Circulation

The patient's circulation should be assessed using a look, listen and feel approach.

Heart rate and rhythm   The patient's radial pulse should be palpated and the heart rate for one full minute noted. During this time the rhythm of the heart rate (regular verses irregular) and the strength of the heart rate should be assessed.

Peripheral temperature   The nurse should also comment upon the patient's peripheral temperature as if this is cold/clammy it may indicate that the patient is compensating for some form of shock **(hypovolaemia**/cardiogenic). If the patient is hot/sweaty it may indicate sepsis or another form of distributive shock (anaphylaxis/**neurogenic shock**). It is also useful to assess **capillary refill** time—normal refill time is less than 2 seconds and any increase in capillary refill time may indicate a sluggish circulation.

> ! *Note*: The assessment of capillary refill and peripheral temperature cannot be recorded when using a simulation manikin. Some centres will supply this information verbally (but only if you request this detail). You are reminded to ask the examiner for the capillary refill time and also whether the patient is cool/clammy or hot and sweaty.

Blood pressure This should be recorded using either a manual or an electric blood pressure device (see Fig. 12.1d). You should give consideration to the systolic pressure, diastolic pressure and changes in **pulse pressure** (difference between systolic and diastolic pressure). Changes in these recordings may help indicate what is happening with the patient. An example of this is that an increasing diastolic pressure and narrowing pulse pressure could indicate the early stages of hypovolaemia because of **compensatory mechanisms.**

Fluid balance   This will have a profound effect on cardiovascular status so you should consider the current fluid balance of the patient (positive/neutral/negative) and report the findings and likely consequence of the findings. Urine output should also be analysed and you should observe for increases or decreases in urine output (see Fig. 12.1e). If urine output is decreased you should calculate the expected output using the formula:

Output per hour = 0.5 ml per kg per hour

Reduced urine output may indicate that the kidneys are not being adequately perfused due to poor cardiac output. If the patient is not catheterized bladder scanning to estimate output may be advised or you may wish to consider urinary catheterization. Again this will not be feasible in

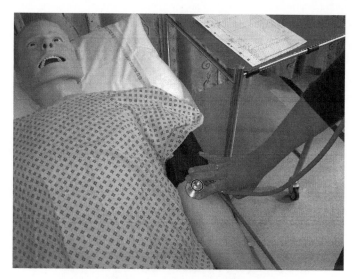

Figure 12.1d An electric blood pressure device

simulation but you may be expected to articulate potential solutions to estimation of urine output.

Temperature   This should be recorded. In some manikins the temperature will be displayed on the bedside monitor. The patient should be observed for signs of infection (temperature above 38.5°C) or signs of hypothermia (temperature below 35.5°C). The Surviving Sepsis Campaign (2007) highlights the need for urgent attention in patients with temperature above 38.5°C.

Document   Having completed the circulation assessment you should document pulse, blood pressure, temperature and fluid balance on the observation chart.

Check   You should observe for the Portsmouth sign (heart rate above systolic blood pressure) when documenting the observations. This sign indicates that the patient's condition is unstable and urgent attention should be sought.

Having completed the circulation assessment you may wish to consider interventions. These may include:

- Medical emergency team call/**crash team** call if no cardiac output detected.

If the patient has a cardiac output

- Change of position to improve blood pressure (lie patient flat),
- Administration of IV fluids/fluid challenge if prescribed,
- Recording a 12 lead **electrocardiogram (ECG),**
- Adding additional monitoring (ECG, regular BP recordings, continuous saturation monitoring),
- Informing medics and following local guidance in respect of the management of sepsis if temperature is high.

Disability

The term disability is referring to the assessment of neurological status and consideration. Generally in acute situations a crude gauge of neurological status is acceptable and in most situations

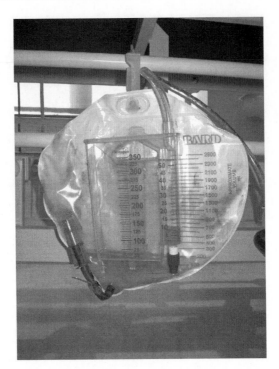

Figure 12.1e Observe for increase or decrease in urine output

the **AVPU** tool will suffice. This is a very simplistic assessment that allows quick evaluation of consciousness levels (Jevons 2007). It is not and should not replace a full neurological examination if the patient's condition requires this.

AVPU stands for:

- **A**lert,
- Responds to **V**oice,
- Responds to **P**ain,
- **U**nconscious.

Resuscitation Council (2006)

Most situations will require you to conduct a formal neurological assessment if the patient responds only to pain or is unconscious. In this group of patients consideration should be given to the patient's ability to maintain their own airway and emergency help may need to be sought.

You should consider factors that might affect the consciousness levels and if there are signs of deteriorating neurological function (the score is V, P or U) you should:

- Record a blood glucose level to assess for hypoglycaemia,
- Review medication chart to note for any administration of medication that may affect consciousness levels, e.g. opiate based analgesia.

It is also appropriate to assess for pain levels in the neurological assessment (see Fig. 12.1f) as worsening pain may indicate deterioration, e.g. haemorrhage within the cranial cavity or raising intracranial pressure (Creed *et al.* 2010).

Document   Having assessed the patient's neurological function you should document the AVPU or Glosgow Coma Score (GCS) if used on an observation chart.

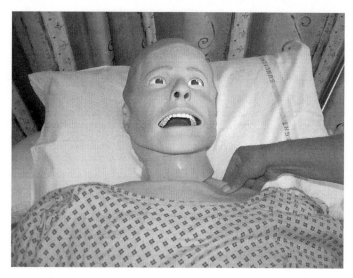

Figure 12.1f Assess for pain levels in neurological assessment

Consideration should be given to:

- Correction of hypoglycaemia if patient's blood glucose is low,
- Maintenance of safety if conscious levels are affected (V or U score),
- Telephoning for an urgent medical review.

Exposure/Everything else/Escalation

Maintaining patient dignity you will be required to remove bed clothing and observe for any obvious causes of the patient's deterioration (Fig. 12.1g). This will include ruling out obvious forms of shock as well as consideration of fluid overload and **deep vein thrombosis/venous thromboembolism (VTE).**

- Hypovolaemia: you should check any wound drains/observe for pooling of blood in the bed. If the patient has a wound consideration should be given to observing the wound site for signs of bleeding/swelling that may indicate blood loss.
- Sepsis: you should observe for flushed appearance alongside decreasing diastolic blood pressure and fast capillary refill time.
- Anaphylaxis: you should note any signs of redness/urticaria, again impossible to simulate but some centres will supply this information verbally but only if you request this detail. You may want to ask the examiner if there are signs of urticaria or redness that may indicate anaphylaxis.
- Deep vein thrombosis/VTE: you should note any calf swelling, pain on inspiration or expectoration of blood as these may indicate development of a pulmonary embolism, again impossible to simulate but some centres will supply this information verbally but only if you request this detail. You may want to ask the examiner if the calf appears swollen/red/painful.
- Fluid overload: you should observe for any signs of dependent oedema. This may be found on feet, ankles, hands, wrist or on the sacral area. Again impossible to simulate but some centres will supply this information verbally but only if you request this detail. You may want to ask if there are signs of dependent oedema.

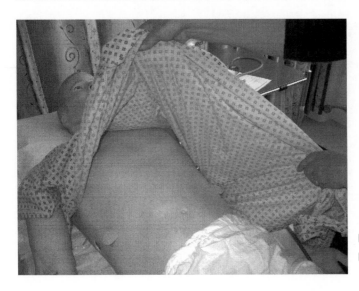

Figure 12.1g Exposure of patient

Document   Having completed **exposure** you should document changes and it may be helpful to review documentation to explore:

- Trends from observation (fast or slow deterioration),
- Review of any tests, e.g. blood results, 12 lead ECG,
- Anything that may impact on the patient's condition.

It is useful to allow some time to step back and consider changes and potential consequences of all of the patient's changes (see Fig. 12.1h).

Calculation of track and trigger score

The nurse should calculate the track and trigger score if this is being used. Once this is complete the nurse should then ensure appropriate escalation. The track and trigger score will generally indicate the degree of deterioration. If the score is low it may only necessitate increasing the frequency of observations. If the score is high then urgent attention should be sought and escalation policies followed.

It is probably advisable to follow the NICE (2007) guidance on escalation unless a local policy is available and you may be expected to articulate who you would call and provide rationale for this. The guidance suggests:

- **Low score/concern.** Patients scoring low scores should have the frequency of their observations increased as a matter of course and the nurse in charge informed.
- **Medium score/concern.** Where patients score medium scores areas of concern should be escalated to the primary medical team wherever possible. Outreach could also be contacted if this service is available.
- **High score/concern.** Where the patient's score is high there should be immediate escalation of concern to an appropriate team. This may include medical emergency teams, outreach calls, anaesthetists and cardiac arrest teams. The urgency of this escalation should be articulated clearly and the need for an immediate response stressed (see Fig. 12.1i).

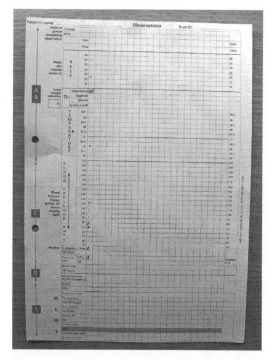

Figure 12.1h Review observations and consider all changes

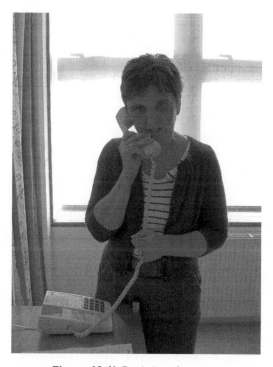

Figure 12.1i Escalation of concern

Communication It is likely that you will be assessed on your ability to hand over your concerns to the nurse in charge or the doctor. In some simulations you will have a telephone and be able to ring an examiner acting as a 'medic'.

 KEY POINT! It is likely that your ability to communicate your concerns succinctly and in a logical manner will be assessed and this may, to an extent, be one of the most difficult parts of the assessment. You are reminded to use a systematic tool such as the SBAR (see earlier section on communication). A confident approach is useful in this area of assessment.

 To help you prepare for the OSCE please go to our website where you can listen to a nurse communicating her concerns to a medic over the phone. Note how she does this succinctly yet uses SBAR to provide all the necessary details.

☑ **Putting it all together!**

As stated earlier this is clearly quite a complex skill to master and so Box 12.2 provides a useful recap of all aspects of this skill.

Box 12.2 **Putting it all together: systematic assessment of the acutely ill patient**

1. Introduce yourself to the patient,

2. Gain consent where able,

3. Airway:
   - Is patient talking to you?
   - Any signs of obstruction?
   - Any abnormal noises?
   - Is there silence?
   - Do you need airway adjuncts?
   - Any laboured breathing/paradoxical breathing indicative of obstruction?

4. Breathing:
   - Rate,
   - Rhythm,
   - Depth,
   - Abnormal pattern,
   - Symmetry,
   - Effort,
   - Use of accessory muscles,
   - Presence of cyanosis.

5. Circulation
   Heart rate:
   - Strength,
   - Speed,
   - Rhythm,
   - Regularity.

Blood pressure:
- Systolic pressure,
- Diastolic pressure,
- Pulse pressure.

6. Temperature:
- Hot/cold,
- Peripheral temperature: cool/clammy/delayed capillary refill.

7. Other factors
- How does patient feel? Patient tells you, e.g. 'I don't feel well',
- Chest pain.

8. Assessment of fluid status
- Fluid balance (needs to be up to date and accurate),
- Urine output,
- Any signs of fluid overload/dehydration.

9. Disability
Neurological factors
- AVPU,
- Blood glucose,
- Analgesia,
- Medication,
- Pain score.

10. Exposure/Everything else/Escalation
Exposure: Maintain dignity but expose patient (look under sheets/clothing)
- Any signs of bleeding?
- Any signs of fluid loss?
- Any oedema/where is this?
- Any signs of sepsis?
- Any signs of DVT/VTE?
- Any rashes?

Everything else:
- Recent blood results,
- Full history,
- Identify trends,
- Review ECG if appropriate,
- Step back and consider everything that may impact on patient through fresh eyes.

Escalation:
- Follow escalation policy on track and trigger chart,
- Call outreach/MET/Medic.
- Use SBAR tool:
  - Situation: where are you/who are you/why calling?
  - Background: PMH (past medical history), reason for admission, summary treatment to date.
  - Assessment: use ABCDE framework, hand over findings systematically. State your concern. Articulate any suspicions.
  - Recommendation: what do you want doctor/outreach/team to do? Clarify an action plan and document this clearly.

Examiners' marking criteria

Various tools will be utilized to assess your competence at recognizing and responding to acute deterioration. As stated in earlier chapters it is advisable to review your own university's marking criteria. An example of marking criteria is included in Table 12.1.

Table 12.1 **Example of examiners' marking criteria**

Student's name and cohort year	
Expected performance criteria	Demonstrated Yes/No
Decontaminates hands.	
Proceeds in a calm manner.	
Approaches the patient in a professional manner and introduces self.	
Communicates with patient throughout the assessment.	
Explains the need for assessment and gains consent, where able.	
Assesses **A**irway for patency: • Observation for visual signs of obstruction, • Observation for auditory signs of obstruction, • Observation for presence of air movement (places hand or face near patient's mouth). Appropriate action is taken to include: • Change in patient's position, • Airway adjunct insertion, • Oxygen.	
Assesses **B**reathing and is able to comment upon: • Rate, • Rhythm, • Depth, • Pattern, • Symmetry, • Use of accessory muscles, • Patient's colour, • Any additional respiratory sounds, • Ability to cough effectively. Appropriate action is taken to include: • Position change, • Administration of oxygen, • Saturation monitoring.	

Table 12.1 (*continued*)

Student's name and cohort year	
Expected performance criteria	Demonstrated Yes/No

Assesses **C**irculation and is able to comment upon:
  • Pulse,
  • Heart rate and rhythm,
  • Regularity of pulse,
  • Blood pressure
    (systolic/diastolic/pulse pressure),
  • Tactile signs, e.g. peripherally cool,
  • Capillary refill time,
  • IV access,
  • Urine output.
 	
Appropriate action is taken to include:
  • IV access if not already available,
  • Instigates cardiac monitoring,
  • 12 lead ECG,
  • Reporting to doctor/senior nurse/outreach.	

Assesses for **D**isability and is able to demonstrate:
  • AVPU,
  • GCS if required,
  • Need for blood glucose monitoring,
  • Assessment of pain,
  • Review of analgesia.
 	
Appropriate action is taken if depressed level of consciousness to include:
  • Repositioning patient
    (lateral position),
  • Remains with patient at all times,
  • Completes neurological assessment if required.	

Is able to assess **E**xposure and demonstrate:
  • Maintenance of privacy,
  • Observation for signs of injury/haemorrhage,
  • Signs of fluid loss,
  • Assessment of lower limbs (oedema/swelling),
  • Assessment for rashes/urticaria,
  • Any signs of sepsis,
  • Analysis of results charts,
  • Calculates the track and trigger score.	

Is able to explain the situation to the patient.	
Is able to summarize findings to examiner. Calls for help: can hand over to the doctor using SBAR principles.	

Examiners' questions

Some universities may assess your knowledge in relation to assessment of acute deterioration and it is useful to prepare for that if that is a requirement. Some typical questions are included in Box 12.3.

Box 12.3 Example of examiners' questions

1. Which groups of patients may be prone to deterioration?
2. Which groups of patients may have airway problems?
3. Which observation will alter first?
4. Why does respiration change if patient is deteriorating?
5. What else do you need to consider alongside oxygen saturations and why?
6. What is the significance of the systolic and diastolic blood pressure?
7. Why is it useful to examine the pulse pressure?
8. Why do patients develop tachycardia
9. Which groups of patients may become bradycardic?
10. What are the common causes of hypovolaemic shock?
11. How might the patient present in the compensatory stage of hypovolaemic shock?
12. How might the patient present in the progressive stage of shock?
13. How might sepsis present?

Answers are provided at the end of the chapter.

✗ Common errors at this station

This is quite a stressful station to undertake and a number of errors occur; these include problems related to failure to:

- Introduce yourself/communicate with the simulation manikin,
- Maintain infection control measures,
- Gain consent for patient assessment,
- Check patient's airway or articulate that you are checking airway,
- Explain what you are checking and why,
- Assess the patient systematically,
- Include all elements of assessment,
- Respond appropriately to any changes you find,
- Complete all of assessment before escalating concern to the doctor (except in clear emergency scenarios),
- Step back and appropriately review the situation,

- Understand the significance of your assessment findings,
- Demonstrate ability to seek appropriate help.

Alongside these, other common errors include:

- Panicking and becoming stressed,
- Rushing handover,
- Incoherent handover,
- Poor communication of concern,
- Poor timing in the station/running out of time.

✚ Top tips for passing this station

Care should be taken at this station to avoid the common pitfalls. However, if you do make a mistake you could consider the following:

- Returning to areas that you have missed as you will still be awarded points for this even if it is out of sequence.
- Suggesting additional treatment/assessments at the end of the exam if you feel that you have missed something.
- Providing explanation regarding your actions at the end of the exam if you forgot during the exam itself.

The key to passing this exam station is demonstrating the ability to:

- Follow a systematic approach,
- Remain calm,
- Conduct a thorough assessment,
- Summarize your findings,
- Ensure appropriate escalation,
- Communicate changes effectively.

You may enhance your ability to pass this station by practising this skill and there are several things that students have found helpful:

- Practising alongside your colleagues in clinical skills room,
- Attending university practice and theory sessions,
- Using the skill in practice with your mentor and asking for constructive feedback,
- Working a day with a critical care outreach practitioner to observe experts using this skill,
- Attending study sessions that are run in practice (if the NHS Trust allows this),
- Practising sequence whilst being timed; this allows you to roughly calculate how much time is needed for each part of the assessment.

To help you practise this we have provided a fictional example of a deteriorating patient online for you to use. Print this off and in a group of three:

- One can be the examiner and can walk through the sequence,
- One can read out instructions and respond when asked by the examinee,
- One can use the examiner's marking sheet to give feedback.

Box 12.4 **A student's view**

'I found this station quite frightening at first because there was so much to remember. Remembering the ABC format helped loads and I attended the practice sessions and tried, as best I could to practise in my ward. I was glad it was a formative assessment but I learnt so much from the assessment and I know this has built my confidence for handling emergencies in clinical practice when I am qualified.'

Third year student nurse after a formative OSCE assessment

 Online resource centre

To help you prepare for the OSCE please go to our website where you can listen to a nurse communicating her concerns to a medic over the phone; note how she does this succinctly yet uses SBAR to provide all the necessary details. Go to **www.oxfordtextbooks.co.uk/orc/caballero/**.
Demonstration of systematic assessment is also available online at
www.oxfordtextbooks.co.uk.orc/caballero/.

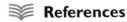 **References**

British Thoracic Society (2008). *Guideline for Emergency Oxygen Use in Adult Patients*. London: BTS.

Creed, F., Dawson, J. and Looker, K. (2010). Assessment tools and track and trigger scoring systems. In: Creed, F., and Spiers, C. (2010) *Care of the Acutely Ill Adults: An Essential Guide for Nurses*. Oxford: Oxford University Press.

Cretikos, M., Bellamo, R., Hillman, K., Chen, J., Finfer, S. and Flabouris, A. (2008). Respiratory rate as an indicator of acute illness. *Medical Journal of Australia*, 188(11): 657–659.

Department of Health (2009). *Competencies for Recognising and Responding to Acutely Ill Adults in Hospital. Draft Guidelines for Consultation*. London: DOH, HMSO.

Endacott, R., Jevon, P. and Cooper, S. (2009). *Clinical Nursing Skills: Core and Advanced*. Oxford: Oxford University Press.

Jevon, P. (2007). *Treating the Critically Ill Patient*. Oxford: Blackwell Publishing.

McGloin, H., Adam, S.K. and Singer, M. (1999). Unexpected deaths and referrals to intensive care of patients on general wards: are some potentially avoidable? *Journal of the Royal College of Physicians*, 33: 255–259.

McQuillan, P., Pilkington, S. and Allan, A. (1998). Confidential enquiry into quality of care before admission to intensive care. *British Medical Journal* 316: 1853–8.

National Confidential Enquiry into Patient Outcome and Death (2005). *An Acute Problem?* London: NCEPOD.

National Patient Safety Agency (2007). *Safer Care for the Acutely Ill Patient: Learning from Serious Incidents*. London: NPSA.

NHS Institute for Innovation and Improvement (2008). *No Delays Achiever, Service Improvement Tools (SBAR)*. London: NHS.

NICE (2007). *Acutely Ill Patients in Hospital: Recognition of and Response to Acute Illness of Adults in Hospital*. London: HMSO.

Resuscitation Council (2006). *Advanced Life Support*, 5th edn. London: Resuscitation Council.

Smith, G. (2003). *ALERT: Acute Life Threatening Events, Treatment and Recognition*. 2nd edn. Portsmouth: University of Portsmouth.

Surviving Sepsis Campaign (2007). www.survingsepsis.org.

Appendix: answers to examiners' questions

1. Any patient's condition may deteriorate at any time and the nurse should be vigilant for change in all patients. Those patients who are at particular risk include:
    *   The elderly,
    *   The very young,
    *   Those with pre-existing condition,
    *   Malnourished patients,
    *   Cancer patients,
    *   Post operative patients.

2. Any patient but again those particularly at risk include:
    *   Post operative patients,
    *   Patients who are drowsy,
    *   Patients on large doses of opiate based analgesia,
    *   Patients admitted with acute neurological problems, e.g. head injury or stroke,
    *   Those patients with pre-existing neurological problems,
    *   Those patients with new or evolving neurological disease.

3. Respiration will change before any other sign.

4. The need for more oxygen is apparent in any situation of patient deterioration. The respiratory drive will therefore automatically increase in an attempt to increase oxygenation.

5. Saturation recordings need to be reviewed in line with oxygen requirements as this gives an indication of how poor the patient's oxygenation actually is. For example, if a patient has saturations of 90% on air there is scope to improve oxygenation by adding supplementary oxygen. However, if a patient has saturations of 90% on 15 litres of oxygen via a non re-breathe mask there is no scope to add more oxygen and that patient is very sick.

6. Systolic and diastolic pressures should be reviewed together as this will give the nurse an idea if the patient is compensating for any form of shock. It would be expected that diastolic changes would be seen before systolic pressure changes. In hypovolaemic and cardiogenic shock, the diastolic pressure would rise; this signifies the release of vasoactive substances that cause vasoconstriction in the compensatory stage of shock. When compensation fails the systolic pressure will rapidly deteriorate. In the early stages of distributive shock the diastolic pressure will fall and systolic pressure may remain constant or fall. Exploration of these pressures may help the nurse to try to identify where the problem is, e.g. bleeding verses sepsis.

7. The pulse pressure is an important indicator of shock and may help the nurse identify whether compensation is occurring. Examination of the pulse pressure will help the nurse to identify whether vasoconstriction or vasodilatation is occurring. In hypovolaemic and cardiogenic shock the pulse pressure will narrow. In sepsis and other forms of distributive shock the pulse pressure will widen as vasodilatation is occurring.

8. Patients develop tachycardia in response to the stimulation of the sympathetic nervous system. In stress responses the parasympathetic nervous system is inhibited (this prevents vagal stimulation to the sino-atrial node and increases the heart rate). At the same time a release of adrenalin acts on the beta receptors in the heart. This increases the heart rate and contractility of the cardiac muscle in an attempt to increase blood pressure. Some patients who are deteriorating may also develop cardiac rhythm problems that result in tachycardia, e.g. atrial fibrillation/supra ventricular tachycardia.

9. Patients with cardiac problems, e.g. right sided myocardial infarctions and patients with heart block, may develop bradycardia. Additionally patients with hypothermia, raised intracranial pressure, neurogenic shock and hypothyroidism may become bradycardic. Caution is advised in patients who are beta blocked as they may not exhibit raising heart rate in response to shock conditions.

10. Common causes include:
    *   Excessive blood loss,
    *   Loss of body fluids,

- Movement of fluid into another space (third space),
- Dehydration,
- Excessive diuretics,
- Burns,
- Vomiting/diarrhoea.

11. In the compensatory stages of shock the patient will present with:
    - Increased respiratory rate,
    - Tachycardia,
    - Normal or slightly raised systolic pressure,
    - Increasing diastolic pressure,
    - Narrowing pulse pressure,
    - Increased capillary refill time,
    - Cool peripheries.

12. In the progressive stage of shock the patient will present with:
    - Hypotension,
    - Tachycardia,
    - Increased respirations,
    - Pallor,
    - Sweating,
    - Decreased levels of consciousness,

13. Sepsis will usually present with:
    - Increased temperature,
    - Increased respiratory rate,
    - Tachycardia,
    - Warm peripheries,
    - Quick capillary refill times (less than 2 seconds),
    - Patient reporting feeling 'fluey',
    - Increased white cell count,
    - Increased C reactive protein,
    - Increased blood lactate.

Patients with neutropenia may not present with typical pyrexia
Patients in late stages of sepsis may present with hypothermia.

Chapter 13

Basic life support (BLS)

Clare Cree

◎ Chapter aims

This chapter will enable you to:

- Revise key material in relation to BLS,
- Follow a step by step guide to BLS,
- Understand how to prepare and revise for this OSCE,
- Highlight common problems at this station and identify how these may be avoided.

▶ Introduction

This chapter will focus on preparing you to undertake an OSCE in the skill of basic life support (BLS), in a cardiac arrest situation, following the Resuscitation Council (UK) Guidelines (2010). Basic life support guidance is aimed especially at adults who in their professions have a duty to respond to a cardiac arrest. Basic life support refers to maintaining the airway, breathing and circulation without the use of any equipment, other than protective devices (Resuscitation Council (UK) 2010). A number of studies (Ahmet and Sarac 2009; Berdowski *et al.* 2009; Oermann *et al.* 2011) recognize that effective implementation of guidance is likely to be enhanced by comprehensive and timely education. Soar *et al.* (2010) suggest that survival from cardiac arrest is dependent on a number of factors—particularly that respondents are well equipped and practiced in the skill and that quality educational packages are readily available to those responders. This chapter will endeavour to provide you with the relevant information to revise the components required to complete an OSCE in the skill. Emphasis is placed on the importance of providing effective, good quality chest compressions whilst minimizing any pauses and so maximizing blood flow and oxygenation.

📖 Key revision for your simulated examination

❗ *Note:* The first aspect of the BLS skill you will be expected to carry out during your OSCE is a full risk assessment of the situation including safety and infection control issues. ❗

Safety

A respondent to any medical emergency should not put themselves or those around them at any risk. If this is impossible, however, measures should be taken to minimize that risk whilst ensuring no further harm comes to the casualty. In your OSCE, you will be expected to review the surrounding area for hazards, e.g. deep water, electricity, oncoming vehicles, fire and smoke, falling debris, biological threats, etc., to ensure your own and the patient's safety.

> ! *Note:* This will depend on the way in which your OSCE station has been set up and if there ! are no threats to yourself or the patient you will need to verbalize to the examiner that you have checked the surrounding area and that it is safe for you to continue.

Only if the casualty or respondent is at risk of significant further injury should they be moved to a safe place. Moving the casualty, however, should not propose any injury to the respondent.

> ! *Note:* It is highly unlikely that you would be expected to move the patient during this OSCE ! but still be prepared to if this will be required.

Particularly in the health care environment it is necessary to protect the casualty, respondent/s and other patients or clients from infective hazards and for this reason personal protective equipment (PPE) is available in the form of disposable gloves, aprons, goggles, masks and hand decontamination either in gel form or washing facilities. Should your scenario be a hospital based cardiac arrest you will be expected to decontaminate your hands and put on gloves and apron prior to commencing BLS.

> ! *Note:* All the necessary personal protective equipment will be made available to you at the ! OSCE station.

Health care workers and patients are vulnerable to communicable diseases due to their highly contagious nature and the close proximity of the population within the environment (Rothman *et al.* 2006). Studies following the severe acute respiratory syndrome (SARS) epidemic in 2003 (Chan-Yeung 2004; Chen *et al.* 2004) showed that outbreaks of infection occur rapidly when health care workers are overstretched. It is when situations are at their most stressful that health care workers must follow the most basic of infection control principles during all patient contact to minimize the spread of unknown pathogens into the general community.

> ✱ KEY POINT! Once the safety of the casualty, you as the respondent and those around you has been secured you can commence the basic life support algorithm (Fig. 13.1a).

The Resuscitation Council (UK) has developed an **algorithm** demonstrating the sequence in which events should occur. This algorithm will now be gone through step by step to guide you through your OSCE.

Responsiveness

In order to check for responsiveness you will be expected to gently shake the casualty's shoulders and ask loudly, 'Are you alright?' as demonstrated in Fig. 13.1b.

If the casualty makes a response you should try to find out what is wrong with them so that this can be relayed to any help that is summoned. The casualty should be checked regularly for any signs of deterioration.

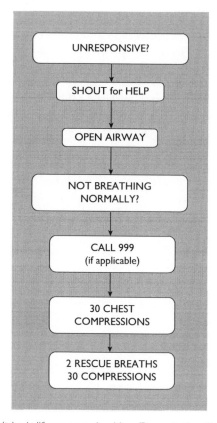

Figure 13.1a Adult basic life support algorithm (Resuscitation Council (UK) 2010).

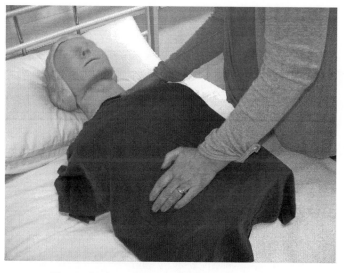

Figure 13.1b Check for responsiveness

If the casualty does not make any response to the 'shake and shout', help should be summoned immediately. If you are alone with the casualty and there is no response to your call for help you should open the airway and confirm absence of normal breathing before leaving your casualty to summon help.

! *Note:* As this is an OSCE to assess your competency in this skill the casualty will not respond ! and you will be expected to put out an emergency call once you have established an unresponsive casualty. This call could be a shout, 2222 call in a hospital or 999 call outside of a hospital. Some OSCE stations may have a telephone available for you to do this or you may be required to ask someone else to put the call out. Please make sure you understand what is expected of you in relation to this before commencing the OSCE. You will be assessed for your ability to stay calm, act professionally and communicate clearly throughout this station.

Calling for help

The method for calling for help will be dependent on the individual circumstances. Regardless of the situation help should be sought ultimately from someone who is qualified and capable of providing advanced life support.

In the health care environment this will generally involve pulling an emergency alarm and making a telephone call, or asking someone else to do it, to summon the cardiac arrest or medical emergency team. Each university will have slightly differing protocols for summoning emergency help and therefore it is important that you know what will be expected of you for the OSCE.

! *Note:* Whilst you are waiting for help to arrive you will be expected to open the casualty's ! airway.

Opening the airway

Basic life support follows the 'ABC' method of assessment and treatment advocated for all medical emergencies (NICE 2007). 'A' is for airway and it is important to open this before moving on to any further treatment or assessment. Without an intact airway it will be impossible for the casualty to take in oxygen. The longer the organs and tissues, especially the brain, are without oxygen the less likely the casualty is to recover without any long term damage.

There are two methods for ensuring the casualty's airway is open. Firstly the preferred 'head tilt chin lift' method and secondly the 'jaw thrust' are techniques that will minimize further damage where spinal injury is suspected. The jaw thrust is not recommended for the untrained rescuer to perform as it is difficult to learn and execute effectively (Resuscitation Council (UK) 2010).

! *Note:* You will not be expected to demonstrate a 'jaw thrust' in your OSCE. !

To do the 'head tilt chin lift' effectively, the casualty should be placed on their back. You will kneel next to the casualty, placing one hand on the victim's forehead, and gently tilt the head backwards.

Using two fingertips of the other hand, place them under the casualty's chin and lift the chin to open the airway (Fig. 13.1c). During the assessment of airway it is important to check that there are no foreign bodies or sputum or vomit obstructing the airway. If these are present they should be removed, using suction if required. Once the airway has been opened you must then check for signs of normal breathing.

Signs of normal breathing

Looking for signs of normal breathing should be done for a time not exceeding 10 seconds with the airway open. Therefore you must maintain the position described previously whilst checking whether there is any chest movement, breath sounds or air coming from the casualty's mouth. This is best done when you remain in a kneeling position, placing your cheek just above the casualty's mouth and nose, and utilize a look, listen and feel approach to assess for breathing.

Small, infrequent and noisy gasps of breath may be evident from the casualty during a cardiac arrest situation. In fact, Bobrow *et al.* (2008) describe these as 'agonal gasps' and suggest that they are common in as many as 40% of cases. This, however, must not be confused with normal breathing and should not delay commencement of the next step in the algorithm. If you are in any doubt you should act as if there is no normal breathing (Ewy 2007) and begin chest compressions.

Note: During the OSCE your casualty will not have any breathing sounds so you will need to move onto the next step of the algorithm. If you have not already summoned help you should call for help. This call could be a 2222 call in a hospital or 999 call outside of a hospital.

Thirty chest compressions

Chest compressions should be started without delay and you will be expected to give 30 chest compressions without interruption. Early chest compressions will improve the casualty's potential for survival and prognosis (Resuscitation Council (UK) 2010).

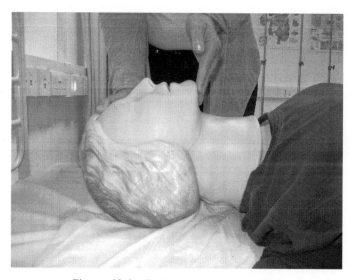

Figure 13.1c The 'head tilt chin lift' method

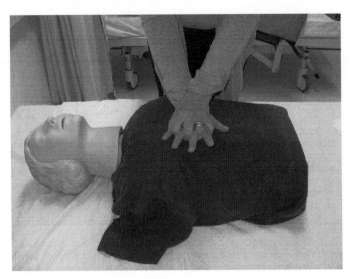

Figure 13.1d Correct hand position for performing chest compression

Figure 13.1d demonstrates the correct hand position for performing chest compressions. You should be kneeling beside the casualty with the heel of one hand in the centre of the casualty's chest. The heel of the other hand should be placed on top of the first hand and the fingers should be interlocked to ensure pressure is not exerted over the ribs, abdomen or the end of the sternum (breastbone). You should then position yourself vertically to the casualty's chest with your arms straight. A downward pressure should then be applied quickly and released. It should be aimed to depress the casualty's chest between 5 and 6 cm in depth at a rate of 100–120 compressions per minute whilst allowing the chest to recoil completely after each compression (Resuscitation Council (UK) 2010).

! *Note:* Some manikins used during OSCEs will have a digital display unit which will be able to provide you and the examiner with visual feedback on how effective your chest compressions are and if your hands are in the correct position. Make sure you are familiar with this technology if it is going to be used in your OSCE.

Compressions should be repeated 30 times consecutively without interruption. You will find it easier to count each compression (you can do this out loud during the OSCE and this is positively encouraged) in order to recognize the number performed and it should be recognized that delivering chest compressions effectively can be exhausting. Zhan *et al.* (2009) studied the effects of two different methods of counting on rescuer fatigue during cardiac arrest, ascertaining that counting from 1–10 three times was less tiring, it taking longer for the respondents to reach peak heart rate than when counting from 1–30 continuously. They suggest this is due to the polysyllabic nature of the numbers counted in the continuous count.

 KEY POINT! When 30 continuous chest compressions have been delivered you can then progress to the final step on the resuscitation algorithm.

Two rescue breaths: Thirty compressions

Once 30 chest compressions have been delivered you will be expected to deliver two breaths via the casualty's mouth in an attempt to inflate the lungs so that further oxygen may be delivered to the system during the next round of compressions. The casualty's airway should be opened again in order to deliver effective **rescue breaths.**

In a health care environment masks should be available with a one-way valve to assist in the delivery of the rescue breaths (Fig. 13.1e). Larger 'bag-mask' devices that can also be connected to a supplemental oxygen supply may also be available although this piece of equipment requires two people to operate it effectively (Fig. 13.1f).

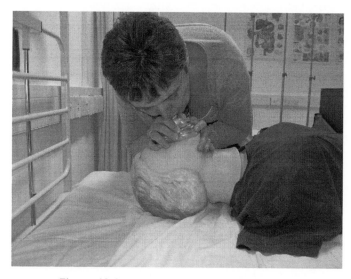

Figure 13.1e One-way valve environmental mask

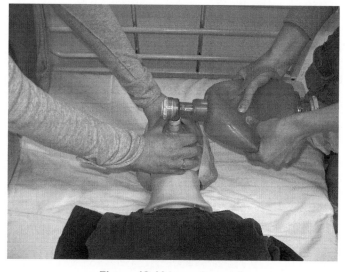

Figure 13.1f Larger bag-mask

! *Note:* All relevant masks will be made available to you at the OSCE station. !

You will now be expected to carry out rescue breaths utilizing the following process in order:

- The student opens the casualty's airway.
- The student closes the casualty's nose by gently pinching the soft area of the casualty's nose with the index finger and thumb of one hand.
- The student allows the casualty's mouth to open whilst still maintaining the 'chin lift' position.
- The student places their mouth over the casualty's mouth ensuring there can be no leakage of air between the contact.
- The student blows steadily into the casualty's mouth whilst watching the casualty's chest rise.
- The student takes their mouth away from the casualty's and watches the chest fall.
- The student repeats the process again.

You should make no more than two attempts at giving effective rescue breaths because further attempts would increase the time in which the casualty has no circulating blood being delivered to the tissues. These two breaths should not take longer than 5 seconds.

Once this process has been completed you will be expected to begin giving 30 chest compressions in exactly the same manner as in the previous step on the algorithm. This part of the algorithm will continue until either qualified help arrives or the victim begins to show signs of regaining consciousness or the examiner asks you to stop. It is vital that there is no time delay in beginning subsequent sets of chest compressions associated with the delivery of rescue breaths as in fact chest compressions alone may be more beneficial than any unproductive pause. Soar *et al.* (2010) actually suggest that in some circumstances it can be as effective to give continual chest compressions without pausing to deliver rescue breaths at all. They do recommend, however, that personnel with a 'duty to care' (which you are) should be trained to do chest compressions and ventilations.

Delivery of chest compressions and rescue breaths at a ratio of 30:2 will continue until the examiner asks you to stop.

! *Note:* In a real clinical situation in order to reduce fatigue it may be necessary for others to take ! over chest compressions at regular intervals although pauses should be kept to an absolute minimum. If someone is to recover from a cardiac arrest the aim of the respondent/s should be that the casualty will be of full mental capacity when they do eventually regain consciousness or no worse than they were prior to the incident. To achieve this a respondent must provide optimum artificial circulation and ventilation.

! *Note:* Some OSCEs on BLS might expect you to demonstrate your ability to put someone into ! the **recovery position** at the end of the scenario; please follow the directions on how to do this.

Recovery position

If the casualty is breathing normally they should be moved into the recovery position and their breathing closely monitored until help arrives. The following sequence is recommended by the Resuscitation Council (UK) to achieve the recovery position:

- Kneel by the casualty, making sure both their legs are straight.
- Place the nearest arm out at right angles from the casualty's body with the elbow bent up toward the head and palm of the hand facing up.

- Bring the furthest arm across the casualty's chest, holding the back of their hand against the near side cheek.
- Bend the far leg at the knee, keeping the foot on the ground.
- The far leg should then be used to lever the casualty onto their side.
- Once on their side, the casualty's upper hip and knee should be manoeuvred so that they are at right angles to each other.
- Tilt the casualty's head back so that the airway remains open.

The OSCE station

The OSCE is likely to be performed in a clinical skills laboratory at your university campus, and you will generally have a time limit of between 10 and 15 minutes to complete the skill. The room will be set up with a manikin either in a bed or on the floor and all relevant equipment will be made available to you, e.g. PPE and masks.

You will be expected to communicate with the manikin and carry out the skill of basic life support following these steps. Following the completion of the procedure you may be asked some questions about basic life support so be prepared!

 Examiners' marking criteria

The criteria used to assess your basic life support skills will vary between universities and will depend on the type of casualty you have. An example of simulated examination criteria are in Table 13.1.

Table 13.1 **Example of examiners' marking criteria**

Student's name and cohort year	
Expected performance criteria	Demonstrated Yes/No
Check that it is safe to approach the casualty.	
Try to get a response from the casualty.	
If no response shout for help (pull emergency buzzer if available).	
Open the airway.	
Look, listen and feel for breathing for no longer then 10 seconds.	
If no breathing present or patient making inadequate respiratory effort ensure 999 or 2222 (or other emergency number) has been called.	
Perform 30 chest compressions, rate 100–120 per minute, depth 5–6 cm.	
Attempt two ventilations (mouth to mouth/nose or other appropriate ventilation device).	
Continue to perform **CPR** at a ratio of 30:2 whilst minimizing any interruptions in chest compressions.	
Continue until qualified help arrives, you become exhausted or casualty shows signs of response.	

Examiners' questions

Some universities may assess your knowledge in relation to resuscitation and it is useful to prepare for that if that is a requirement. Some typical questions are included in Box 13.1.

Box 13.1 Example of examiners' questions

1. Before commencing BLS what is the first thing you must do?
2. What PPPE should you think of using?
3. Give three examples of the types of hazards you need to look out for when securing the scene.
4. In what three ways can you call for help?
5. What does the 'A' stand for in the ABC assessment for BLS?
6. Which method of opening the patient's airway is preferred?
7. How long do you take to look for normal signs of breathing once you have opened the airway?
8. How many chest compressions do you do consecutively?
9. What is the ratio of breaths to chest compressions?
10. If your patient shows signs of improvement and starts to breathe on their own what position can you put them in?

Answers can be found at the end of the chapter.

✗ Common errors at this station

A number of errors occur at this station; these include failure to:

- Ensure that the scene is safe,
- Use appropriate PPE (gloves and aprons in hospital arrest situations),
- Put out an emergency call,
- Open the airway adequately,
- Administer 30 consecutive chest compressions in a timely fashion,
- Position hands correctly for effective chest compressions,
- Compress the chest effectively,
- Quickly provide adequete ventilations, thereby increasing the time away from chest compressions,
- Carry out correct breath to chest compression ratios.

✚ Top tips for passing this station

- Practise as much as you can prior to taking the OSCE utilizing all the practical sessions put on by your university skills team.

- Learn the process off by heart so you do not have to spend valuable time thinking about what to do next.
- Revise the underpinning knowledge in relation to basic life support as you may well be asked questions at the end of the procedure. Please refer to the section on questions in this chapter to guide your revision.
- If during the OSCE you realize that you have not done something or that you are doing it incorrectly DO NOT PANIC—just stop, explain to the examiner what is wrong and start again.
- If you need to start again be aware that you may well be under a time constraint so again DO NOT PANIC—carry out the procedure as best you can.
- If you run out of time you will be referred (i.e. not passed yet!) at this attempt but be assured you will be given at least one more opportunity to pass.
- If you pass CONGRATULATIONS, you have mastered a life saving skill.

Online resource centre

You can find further advice and revision help for your OSCEs by going online now to see **www.oxfordtextbooks.co.uk/orc/caballero/.**

References

Ahmet, O. and Sarac, L. (2009). The effects of different instructional methods on students' acquisition and retention of cardiopulmonary resuscitation skills. *Resuscitation,* 81: 555–561.

Berdowski, J. *et al.* (2009). Time needed for a regional emergency medical system to implement resuscitation guidelines 2005—The Netherlands experience. *Resuscitation,* 80: 1336–1341.

Bobrow, B. *et al.* (2008). Gasping during cardiac arrest in humans is frequent and associated with improved survival. *Circulation,* 118: 2550–2554.

Chan-Yeung, M. (2004). Severe acute respiratory syndrome (SARS) and healthcare workers. *International Journal of Occupational Environmental Health,* 10: 421–427.

Chen, S.Y. *et al.* (2004). Facing an outbreak of highly transmissible disease: problems in emergency department response. *Annals of Emergency Medicine,* 44: 93–95.

Ewy, G. (2007). New concepts of cardiopulmonary resuscitation for the lay public: continuous chest compression CPR. *Circulation,* 116: 1907–1915.

National Institute for Health and Clinical Excellence (2007). *NICE Clinical Guideline 50. Acutely Ill Patients in Hospital: Recognition of and Response to Acute Illness in Adults in Hospital.* London: National Institute for Health and Clinical Excellence.

Oermann, M. *et al.* (2011). Effects of monthly practice on nursing students' CPR psychomotor skill performance. *Resuscitation,* 10: 1016–1022.

Resuscitation Council (UK) (2010). *Resuscitation Council Guidelines 2010* (ed. J.P. Nolan). London: Resuscitation Council (UK). www.resus.org.uk.

Rothman, R., Hsieh, Y. and Yang, S. (2006). Communicable respiratory threats in the ED: tuberculosis, influenza, SARS and other aerosolized infections. *Emergency Medicine Clinics of North America,* 24: 989–1017.

Soar, J. *et al.* (2010). European Resuscitation Council Guidelines for Resuscitation 2010, Section 9. Principles of education in resuscitation. *Resuscitation,* 81: 1434–1444.

Zhan, L., Qing, H. and Yang, M. (2009). The effects of two different counting methods on the quality of CPR on a manikin—a randomized control trial. *Resuscitation,* 80: 685–688.

Appendix: answers to examiners' questions

1. Before commencing BLS what is the first thing you must do?
    - Secure the scene and make sure the environment is safe for both the casualty and yourself.

2. What PPE should you think of using:
    - Masks,
    - Gloves,
    - Aprons,
    - Goggles,
    - Aseptic gel.
    - Secure the scene and make sure the environment is safe for both the casualty and yourself.

3. Give three examples of the types of hazards you need to look out for when securing the scene?
    - Deep water,
    - Electricity,
    - Oncoming vehicles,
    - Fire and smoke,
    - Debris,
    - Biological threats.

4. In what three ways can you call for help?
    - Pull emergency call bell,
    - Telephone hospital emergency number,
    - Ask someone else to put the call out for you.

5. What does the 'A' stand for in the ABC assessment for BLS?
    - Airway.

6. Which method of opening the patient's airway is preferred?
    - Head tilt chin lift.

7. How long do you take to look for normal signs of breathing once you have opened the airway?
    - 10 seconds.

8. How many chest compressions do you do consecutively?
    - 30

9. What is the ratio of breaths to chest compressions?
    - 2:30

10. If your patient shows signs of improvement and starts to breathe on their own what position can you put them in?
    - Recovery position.

PART III

Final preparation

Chapter 14
Reflecting upon your OSCE
Fiona Creed

◎ Chapter aims

This chapter will explore learning from your OSCE experience through the reflective process. It will explore:

- Definitions of reflection,
- Why reflection is important after an OSCE,
- Models available to aid your reflection,
- How you can use reflection to learn from the OSCE experience,
- Using feedback from your OSCE to develop practice,
- Moving forward after your OSCE.

➤ Introduction

Once you have completed your OSCE assessment you will be informed of the outcome of the assessment. This may be on the day, if it is a formative assessment, or sometime afterwards, if it is a summative examination that has to be processed through an examination board. You should be provided with detailed written feedback about your performance at the OSCE and it is useful to review this alongside your recollections of the experience as this will help you to learn from the experience.

Reflection is an important tool to use whether you have been successful or unsuccessful during your OSCE. It is important in nursing that we are able to reflect and learn from both positive and negative experiences.

Some universities may require you to reflect on your OSCE as part of the examination. Again this may be on the day, immediately after your OSCE or a short period afterwards by reviewing a video of your OSCE (the latter normally happening as part of a formative learning process).

What is reflection?

Reflection is not unique to nurses and is something that we do throughout our lives. In everyday terms reflection may be described as an examination of our personal thoughts and actions (Somerville and Keeling 2004).

In nursing you will be encouraged to develop reflective skills to facilitate your learning in the university and in practice this is often referred to as reflective practice and is slightly different to 'everyday reflection'. Indeed throughout your nursing career you will be encouraged to develop reflective practice skills and become a reflective practitioner.

Reflection as a process was first discussed in 1933 by John Dewey who first identified the need to evaluate our experiences and learn from them. In nursing as with most concepts there are a number of definitions of reflection and this can at first appear to be confusing. Simplistically reflection can be defined as a process of examining and exploring an issue that is related to an experience that results in new learning. Therefore reflection refers to a series of steps that you may take to question and explore an experience with the aim of learning from it (Hart 2010). Within health care many models of reflection have been developed to facilitate the reflective process and you may be required to utilize a model by your university (models of reflection will be discussed later in this chapter). Most theorists agree that the reflective process can be used to reflect in two ways:

- Reflection on action,
- Reflection in action.

Schon (1983)

The main difference between these two processes is the time when reflection takes place (Hart 2010).

Reflection on action   This is perhaps the commonest form of reflection in nursing. During this process you are encouraged to carefully rerun through events that have occurred in the past. The main aim of this process is to evaluate your strengths and weaknesses and to develop new strategies for being more effective in the future (Somerville and Keeling 2004). This type of reflection is often referred to as retrospective as it occurs after the event you are reflecting on has taken place.

Most nurses will automatically use this sort of reflection after their OSCE to try to decide what their strengths and areas for improvement were during the examination. Sometimes there is a tendency for students to concentrate upon their mistakes and issues they think they have forgotten during the exam and this is not always helpful.

Some universities may require you to reflect upon your actions (reflecting on action) and may use this reflection to enhance your grade. For example if you forget to gain consent as the student in Box 14.1 did you could identify this in your reflection and explain why consent is important. In some universities an effective reflection on action, in which you discuss any potential errors, may make the difference between a pass and fail grade.

Reflection in action   It is acknowledged that reflection in action generally only occurs with very experienced practitioners and is a much more complex form of reflection (Tate and Sills 2004; Somerville and Keeling 2004). Reflection in action involves exploring and reflecting upon a situation

---

Box 14.1 **Student reflection following an OSCE**

'When I reflected upon my OSCE I realized that I forgot to do things in the skills assessment that I know I should have done. I made a few silly mistakes and felt really embarrassed. The worst mistake was putting a thermometer in the patient's ear without consent. I would never do this in a real situation! I think reflecting upon it I was too anxious and had not really prepared for the examination situation.'

whilst you are actually in the situation. A widely recognized nurse theorist, Benner (1984) suggests that this sort of reflection involves experienced nurses using tacit knowledge (knowledge that is difficult to articulate, such as 'a feeling about something') to help you make a decision about something whilst you are in a situation. For example you are assessing a patient whose condition is deteriorating and when you realize that something is 'not quite right' about that patient you alter the way you are assessing the patient in order to find out what is wrong with the patient.

It is unlikely that you will use reflection in action in your OSCE examination as most theorists link this sort of reflection with experienced rather than student practitioners. Even with experience reflection in action would be difficult in a stressful situation like an examination (Cottell 2007).

Why is reflection important in nursing?

There are a number of reasons why your university encourages you to develop reflective skills:

- Reflection can help you to focus upon the knowledge, skills and behaviour that you will need to develop for effective clinical practice.
- Reflection will help you to identify your personal strengths and areas for improvement. In identifying those areas that you feel require improvement you provide an opportunity for future personal and professional development.
- Reflection will encourage you to become more self aware and encourage you to understand your interactions with others.

Reflection will enable you to learn from your experiences and continually enhance your skills and knowledge—an essential component of life long learning.

Using models to aid reflection

Many universities will encourage you to use a model for your reflection on your OSCE experience. A reflective model provides structure and guidance to your reflection on your OSCE and may be used to help you develop more effective reflective skills. The university may decide which model is useful to guide your reflection and you will be required to use that model or you may choose a model that you feel is most appropriate. There are many models of reflection available and it is beyond the scope of this book to discuss all these. However, you are reminded to discuss reflective models with the OSCE team and find out which models you should use and read around these. Models available include:

- Gibbs' reflective cycle,
- Johns' model for structured reflection,
- Kolb's learning cycle,
- Atkin and Murphy's model of reflection,
- Rolfe's framework for reflective practice.

The example that will be briefly described here is Gibbs (1988) as this is commonly used by nursing students. However, regardless of which model you choose to reflect upon your OSCE there is a common approach that is used in all processes that reflect on situations (Tate and Sill 2004).

The initial stage of reflection will be to return to the experience. During the reflection on your OSCE you will need to return to the situation and remember what happened and explore this. It is important that when you are reflecting you are kind to yourself and view the reflective cycle as something to enhance learning rather than destroy your confidence. In most reflections nurses often concentrate

Box 14.2 **Student reflection on an OSCE**

'In my BP assessment I found out the reason why I had failed and that was because I let the cuff down too quickly and could not really hear the systolic and diastolic pressures properly.'

upon what they have not done or what they have done badly. Whilst this negative approach is very common in nursing reflections and may help your professional development it does sometimes prevent us from focusing upon what we have done well. (An example is included in Box 14.2.)

In this segment of the reflection it is clear the student is focusing upon the negative aspect of the OSCE and not focusing upon the positive aspects of her care such as excellent infection control, effective interpersonal skills and maintenance of patient dignity.

Remember when you return to your OSCE experience try not to focus on the negative elements only.

Once you have recollected your experience, it may be of benefit to use a model to help focus your reflection. Gibbs will be discussed as a tool for reflection upon your OSCE experience. Gibbs (1988) developed his reflective cycle in 1988 and it is a useful and simplistic model that can be used to guide reflection and is shown in Fig. 14.1.

The stages of Gibbs' reflective cycle are described briefly here (it may be useful to refer to this work in more detail if you are not already familiar with it).

Describe Event   This stage encourages returning to the experience and describing it. This stage is vital as it allows you to recollect what happened. It is best to do this as soon after the event as possible so that the memory is still fresh, although you may still forget some aspects of the experience.

Feelings   This stage encourages you to explore your feelings during the situation. It enables you to reflect back upon what you were thinking about and any memories about the situation that you consider to be important.

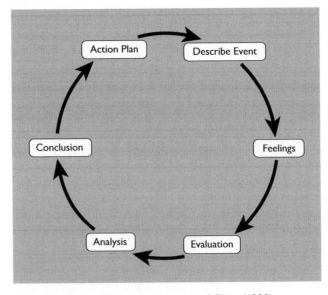

Figure 14.1 Reflective cycle of Gibbs (1988)

Evaluation   This stage encourages you to explore positive and negative aspects of the situation as well as evaluating what happened during the situation.

Analysis   This stage encourages you to break down the situation into its component parts so that you can explore each element separately. During this stage it is important to consider what factors impacted upon the experience.

Conclusion   In this stage you are encouraged to explore the situation from different angles so that you can make your judgement of the situation having explored all the issues that may have been involved in the experience. It may be useful to explore here anything that you feel you handled well or could improve upon.

Action Plan   In this stage you should reflect upon how you would act if you encountered the experience again. You should consider whether you would act differently or whether you would act exactly the same if this situation were repeated. This is an important stage in helping you to summarize learning from the experience.

 When reviewing your own OSCE experience you can use the questions in Box 14.3 to guide your reflection. Do try to complete all of the questions.

 Note you can also download copies of this to print out and write on from our online resource centre: **www.oxfordtextbooks.co.uk/orc/caballero/**.

Box 14.3 **Using Gibbs to reflect upon your OSCE**

1. Describe Event: Describe what happened during your OSCE. Try to remember exactly what happened during the OSCE situation and briefly write it down.

2. Feelings: What were you thinking and feeling at the time of your OSCE? Try to remember how you were feeling. Were you very anxious? Were you calm?

3. Evaluation: List points that were GOOD and BAD about the experience. Try to focus upon positive aspects first. What went well? Was there anything you were pleased about? Once you have fully explored the positive aspects think about any areas you could have improved upon. Try to focus on areas for improvement rather than negatively focus upon 'things you forgot' or 'things that went wrong' as this will help when you come to the action plan stage!

4. Analysis: What sense can you make out of the situation? Break the OSCE situation down into small components and focus on evaluating each of these small parts. Have a number of influences affected your OSCE or was there only one issue?

5. Conclusion: Focus upon answering the following: What went well (remember to celebrate this!)? What could you have done in the OSCE? What perhaps would you not have done in your OSCE?

6. Action Plan: If you had to retake your OSCE again, what would you do differently to ensure you passed? If you have passed your OSCE consider what went well. How will you learn from this experience and remember to repeat this in clinical practice?

Once you have completed this reflective account it is important that you acknowledge the positive outcomes, explore how you can improve and develop an action plan following this experience.

Remember it may take some time getting used to using a structured model of reflection since it encourages us to reflect in much more detail than we are used to in everyday life. Nevertheless it is an important skill to develop as you will be expected to develop your reflective skills throughout your time at university and as a registered nurse!

Making good use of feedback from your OSCE

The focus of discussion has so far emphasized the importance of the development of self reflection during your OSCE and how this can be of benefit to you. However, you are also likely to be provided with some written or verbal feedback from the examiner and it is important that you are able to utilize this and develop the ability to reflect upon feedback from the examiner.

Understandably most students are keen to discover whether they have been successful or unsuccessful with their OSCE and this is of course an important consideration. However, the feedback that you receive, irrespective of your success, can help you to further develop and it is vital that you read and reflect upon feedback as well.

Written or verbal feedback will provide you with an experienced lecturer's opinion regarding your achievement at OSCE and feedback from another perspective is central to the process of reflection (Somerville and Keeling 2004). It is likely that feedback from a lecturer will provide you with an objective opinion of your achievement in your OSCE. Recollect (Chapter 1) that one of the reasons that OSCEs were developed was to provide an objective assessment that provides objective feedback to the student. Your lecturer will highlight areas that you excelled in and areas where there is scope for improvement. It is useful to use this feedback alongside your own personal reflections to develop an action plan following your OSCE.

It may also be of benefit to arrange an appointment with one of your tutors to enable verbal feedback. The tutor may well be able to help coach you with your reflection skills. This will enable you to fully reflect upon the feedback and make an action plan for your own development. Often in the early stages of developing reflective skills it is hard to reflect on feedback and personal experience (Clark 2004). Some students' views on the value of feedback are highlighted in Box 14.4.

Moving forward from your OSCE following success

Whilst achievement at your OSCE will seem like a huge milestone, especially in your first year, it is important that you do not view your OSCE assessment as an end point as you will still have a lot to learn. It is vital that you are able to harness learning from your OSCE and use this for your own professional

---

Box 14.4 Students' views on the value of feedback

Successful student reflecting upon feedback
'It was really nice to get the feedback in the OSCE…it really helped me develop my own practice.'

Unsuccessful student reflecting upon feedback
'There were some skills that I had thought I had passed and when I got the feedback I knew the reason why I had not. I can pick up from this feedback; I have learnt a lot from it.'

development. You can use the experience and feedback to develop an action plan for your future development. You may wish to return to your reflective exercise and begin to highlight your own particular strengths and weaknesses. It may be helpful to split the OSCE into distinct learning areas, e.g. knowledge, skills and professional attributes. In doing this you will be able to see if there are any areas where improvement in knowledge or skills is required. It may be useful to complete the action plan in Table 14.1.

 Note you can also download copies of this to print out and write on from our online resource centre: **www.oxfordtextbooks.co.uk/orc/caballero/**.

What if you are unsuccessful?

Students may initially be unsuccessful at the OSCE. There are a number of reasons for this, some of which have been highlighted throughout the chapters in this book. On some occasions it may be because of failure to prepare; others are unsuccessful because they have become very anxious about the examination and this affects their performance at OSCE. Anxiety is a common issue, as the student's reflection in Box 14.5 highlights.

Bloomfield *et al.* (2010) highlight the need to take time to absorb the information. It may be helpful to view this as a minor setback rather than an endpoint. All universities will allow you at least one more attempt for your OSCE.

Once you have taken time to assimilate the need to retake your OSCE it is important that you prepare for the next attempt at your OSCE. Bloomfield *et al.* (2010) highlight the importance of reflecting on your OSCE experience. It may be useful to focus upon:

- Personal aspects of the OSCE: Did you prepare well, were you excessively anxious, did you forget everything you had learned because you began to panic?
- Knowledge aspects of the OSCE: Did you revise prior to the OSCE? Are there areas that you need to revise in more detail?

Table 14.1 **Action plan following OSCE**

	Strengths	Areas for improvement	Action plan for development
Skill component of OSCE			
Knowledge component of OSCE			
Professional aspects of OSCE			

Box 14.5 **Student reflecting upon anxiety**

'I think the nerves got the better of me. In an exam situation I tend to freeze. I found trying to get normal interaction with my patient in those circumstances really difficult.'

- Skill aspects of the OSCE: Had you practised the skill before? Did you understand how you needed to perform the skill? Do you need to refine your performance of the skill?
- Professional aspect of the OSCE: Did you forget important professional aspects such as consent because it was a simulated environment? Did you feel uncomfortable talking to your 'patient'? Were your interpersonal skills affected by anxiety?

An in-depth personal reflection may enable you to highlight problem areas that you need to address. You may wish to return to your reflective exercise and begin to highlight your own particular strengths and weaknesses. It may be helpful to split the OSCE into distinct learning areas, e.g. knowledge, skills and professional attributes. In doing this you will be able to see if there are any areas where improvement in knowledge or skills is required. It may be useful to complete the action plan in Table 14.1.

When you have completed your reflection and action plan it would be useful to discuss this and perhaps organize some practice sessions with one of the skills lecturers.

 Online resource centre

You can find further advice and revision help for your OSCEs by going online now to see **www.oxfordtextbooks.co.uk/orc/caballero/**.

Box 14.6 Some final reflections from two second year students

Student 1
'I thought the OSCE assessment was good, although a little scary . . . it worked' you could see what you were doing…you did not just fly in and do it like you do in practice, you had to demonstrate knowledge and skills.'

Student 2
'I think that important skills should be examined using an OSCE, because I think if I were a patient and the nurse did not know what she was doing or did not have the knowledge I would be terrified.'

 References

Benner, P. (1984). *From Novice to Expert, Excellence and Power in Clinical Nursing.* California: Addison Wesley.

Bloomfield, J., Pegram, A. and Jones, C. (2010). *How to Pass Your OSCE: A Guide to Success in Nursing and Midwifery.* Harlow: Pearson.

Clark, A. (2004). **Enabling learning through reflective tutorials in the nursing practice setting.** In: Tate, S. and Sills, M. (eds) *The Development of Critical Refection in Health Professionals* Accessed from: www.health.heacademy.ac.uk/publications/.../occasionalpaper04.pdf.

Cottell, P. (2007). A reflection on objective structured clinical examinations (OSCE). *Primary Health Care,* 17(10): 22–23.

Dewey, J. (1933). *How We Think. A Restatement of the Relation of Reflective Thinking to the Educative Process.* Boston: DC Health.

Gibbs, G. (1988). *Learning by Doing: A Guide to Teaching and Learning Methods.* Oxford: Further Education Unit, Oxford Polytechnic.

Hart, S. (2010). *Nursing: Study and Placement Learning Skills*. Oxford: Oxford University Press.

Schon, D. (1983). *The Reflective Practitioner: How Professionals Think in Action*. New York: Basic Books.

Somerville, D. and Keeling, J. (2004). A practical approach to promote reflective practice within nursing. *Nursing Times*, 100(12): 42–46.

Tate, S. and Sills, M. (2004). The development of critical refection in health professionals. Accessed from: www.health.heacademy.ac.uk/publications/.../occasionalpaper04.pdf.

Glossary

Acute Refers to a sudden alteration in the patient's condition, e.g. acute breathlessness, a sudden onset of difficulty breathing.

Affective domain Relates to attitude and professional approach. You will be assessed on this throughout your OSCE.

ALERT© Acute life threatening events, treatment and recognition. This is a well established program used in practice to help identify and treat patients whose condition is deteriorating.

Algorithm A list or set of instructions to solve a problem. In health care the resuscitation algorithm is an important set of instructions that relate to resuscitation processes.

Anaphylaxis An extreme allergic reaction that causes potentially life threatening symptoms in a patient.

Antecubital fossa This is the area on the anterior aspect of the elbow; it contains the tendon of the biceps, the median nerve and the brachial artery. This is the location for auscultation of brachial blood pressure.

Asepsis The absence of any infectious agents such as bacteria, viruses or fungi.

Aseptic technique A non-touch method that minimizes the possibility of cross contamination that could lead to an infection.

Assessment criteria A list of assessment categories that examiners will use to assess you either in clinical practice or in an OSCE.

AVPU A simplistic neurological assessment tool used to provide a quick assessment of neurological status.

Basic life support (BLS) Resuscitation procedures utilized before more advanced life support (utilizing resuscitation equipment) becomes available.

Blood pressure The pressure exerted by the circulating volume on the walls of the blood vessels.

Brachial pulse The pulse from the brachial artery that is situated in the anterior aspect of the elbow (antecubital fossa).

Bradycardia A slower than normal heart rate, usually below 60 beats per minute.

Capillary refill The amount of time for blood to reperfuse an area after blood supply has been artificially reduced by compression. Commonly used to assess circulation by gentle compression of the fingertip for 5 seconds and noting the time taken for blood supply to return. It is usually less than 2 seconds.

Cardiac arrest Cessation of normal circulation of the blood because of failure of the heart to pump effectively.

Carotid pulse The pulse from the carotid artery, situated in the patient's neck.

Catheterization The insertion of a tube. In nursing this is usually into the urethra (urethral catheterization).

Chronic A long term condition.

Cognitive domain Relates to knowledge and understanding. You will be assessed on this throughout your OSCE.

Compensatory mechanism A physiological mechanism that occurs within the body in order to maintain homeostasis. For example the blood vessels may constrict to allow flow of blood to vital organs during episodes of bleeding; this is known as a compensatory reaction.

Contraindication A factor that renders the giving of another medication inadvisable because of the likelihood of reactions.

CPR A technique used to restore circulation and oxygen during periods of cardiac arrest.

Crash team The team who respond following an emergency cardiac arrest call. The team is usually made up of specialist doctors, nurses and other health care professionals.

Deep vein thrombosis The formation of a blood clot in a deep vein. Commonly found in the femoral or popliteal vein.

Diastolic pressure The pressure exerted by the circulating volume on the walls of the blood vessels during relaxation of the ventricles (diastole).

Electrocardiogram (ECG) A graphic recoding of the electrical waveforms from the heart muscle.

Escalation The process of ensuring appropriate referral to a doctor by an experienced nurse during episodes of patient deterioration.

Exposure The final part of the assessment process whereby the patient is fully examined to allow exploration of causes of patient deterioration.

Femoral pulse The pulse from the femoral artery which is located at the top of the leg.

Fluid balance This is normally recorded on a chart representing the total fluid input and output from a patient for 24 hours. The balance refers to the subtraction of the output from the patient's input.

Formative examination An examination designed to provide constructive feedback to a student. This examination does not normally contribute to your overall assessment grade and you may not need to pass this examination.

Hand decontamination Refers to either washing the hands with soap and water or using alcohol gel to prevent cross infection in hospital.

Health care acquired infection An infection acquired at least 72 hours after admission to hospital. Also known as nosocomial infection.

Hypertension Higher than normal blood pressure. Blood pressure is normally considered high if the systolic is 139 mmHg or higher and the diastolic is 90 mmHg or higher.

Hypotension Lower than normal blood pressure. Blood pressure is usually considered hypotensive if the systolic is below 100 mmHg.

Hypothermia Lower than normal body temperature (usually lower than 35.5°C).

Hypovolaemia A low blood volume normally associated with bleeding, severe fluid loss and dehydration.

Indications The reason why a medication is being prescribed.

Infection control The use of several techniques to prevent the spread of infection.

Intramuscular An injection administered into a muscle.

Intravenous An injection administered into a vein.

Korotkoff's sounds The sounds heard via a stethoscope when auscultating blood pressure.

Macroscopic analysis Examination by observation by the human eye.

Manikin A life-like representation of a human used for the purposes of simulation in education, such as SimMan®.

MET team Medical emergency team. A team of doctors and nurses who will respond to acute patient deterioration.

Microscopic analysis Examination by observation by utilizing a microscope, normally performed in a hospital laboratory.

Neurogenic shock A type of shock caused by spinal cord injury which results in failure of the autonomic nervous system to properly regulate sympathetic nervous responses. Patients with this form of shock present with hypotension and bradycardia and are usually warm to touch.

Nosocomial infection Another term for health care acquired infection.

OSCE An examination whereby students are assessed against objective criteria using simulation.

Oxygen saturation The measurement of the amount of oxygen carried bound to the haemoglobin molecule. It is sometimes referred to as SaO_2.

Pathogen An organism that has the ability to cause an infection, e.g. bacteria, viruses, fungi.

Personal protective equipment (PPE) Protective equipment designed to help reduce the spread of infection. PPE includes gloves, aprons, visors, gowns, etc. Local policy normally determines which PPE should be used in each circumstance.

Physiological measurements The recording of measurements that reflect the physiological status of the patient. These normally include blood pressure, pulse, respirations, temperature, oxygen saturations and neurological status.

Popliteal pulse A peripheral pulse located at the back of the patient's knee.

Psychomotor domain Relates to performance of a skill. You will be assessed on this throughout your OSCE.

Pulse Represents the tactile arterial palpation of an artery. It is important to assess the strength of the pulse as it may indicate changes in the patient's condition. For example, a bounding pulse may suggest response to a severe infection whereas a thready weak pulse may represent reduced circulating volume due to bleeding.

Pulse pressure A calculation representing the difference between the systolic and diastolic pressures. A narrowing pulse pressure may indicate haemorrhage whereas a widening pulse pressure may indicate sepsis.

Pyrexia A temperature that is higher than normal, usually above 37.5°C.

Radial pulse A peripheral pulse located in the wrist directly above the thumb.

Reagent strips Chemical strips used in practice to test for the presence of important substances, e.g. urinalysis reagent strips.

Recovery position Refers to the lateral positioning of a patient who is unconscious but has a pulse in order to maintain patient safety until the patient recovers.

Rescue breath An artificial breath used during CPR to maintain oxygenation. It may be mouth to mouth or more commonly mouth to mask.

Respiratory arrest The cessation of spontaneous respiration. It may or may not be accompanied by cardiac arrest.

Sepsis A systemic inflammatory response caused by severe infection.

Shock A failure of the circulatory system to maintain adequate organ perfusion. It may be caused by loss of circulating volume (hypovolaemic shock), failure of the cardiac muscle (cardiogenic shock) or failure of appropriate distribution of the blood supply (distributive shock). Distributive shock includes anaphylaxis, sepsis and neutropenic shocks.

Side effects An adverse or undesirable effect of a medication, e.g. nausea. Common side effects of medications are normally listed in a drugs formulary.

Sphygmomanometers A machine for recording blood pressure. This may be manual or electronic/automated.

Suboptimal care Refers to care that has not reached expected standards. The term suboptimal care is normally used where the patient's deterioration has not been recognized or treated appropriately.

Summative examination An examination that must be passed and which contributes to the overall grade you are awarded.

Systolic pressure The pressure exerted by the circulating volume on the walls of the blood vessels during contraction of the ventricles (systole).

Tachycardia A faster than normal heart beat, normally exceeding 100 beats per minute.

Track and trigger scoring systems A monitoring tool that alerts the user to any abnormality in physiological parameters by firstly tracking the parameters as they are recorded and then triggering a warning if they are outside of the expected range. They are also referred to as early warning scores or modified early warning scores.

Urinalysis The analysis of urine using a chemical reagent strip.

Venous thromboembolism (VTE) A global term that refers to deep vein thrombosis and pulmonary embolism.

Index

Page numbers in *italic* indicate answers to examiners' questions

Printed and bound by CPI Group (UK) Ltd, Croydon, CR0 4YY